Underfed and Overfed

The Global Epidemic of Malnutrition

50

WORLDWATCH PAPER

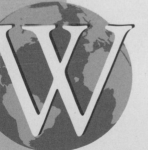

arch
000

Gary Gardner
Brian Halweil

Underfed and Overfed: The Global Epidemic of Malnutrition

GARY GARDNER
AND
BRIAN HALWEIL

Jane A. Peterson, *Editor*

WORLDWATCH PAPER 150

March 2000

THE WORLDWATCH INSTITUTE is an independent, nonprofit environmental research organization in Washington, DC. Its mission is to foster a sustainable society in which human needs are met in ways that do not threaten the health of the natural environment or future generations. To this end, the Institute conducts interdisciplinary research on emerging global issues, the results of which are published and disseminated to decision-makers and the media.

FINANCIAL SUPPORT for the Institute is provided by the Compton Foundation, the Geraldine R. Dodge Foundation, the Ford Foundation, the William and Flora Hewlett Foundation, W. Alton Jones Foundation, Charles Stewart Mott Foundation, the Curtis and Edith Munson Foundation, David and Lucile Packard Foundation, John D. and Catherine T. MacArthur Foundation, Summit Foundation, Turner Foundation, U.N. Population Fund, Wallace Genetic Foundation, Wallace Global Fund, Weeden Foundation, and the Winslow Foundation. The Institute also receives financial support from its Council of Sponsors members—Tom and Cathy Crain, Roger and Vicki Sant, Robert Wallace and Raisa Scriabine, and Eckart Wintzen—and from the many Friends of Worldwatch.

THE WORLDWATCH PAPERS provide in-depth, quantitative and qualitative analysis of the major issues affecting prospects for a sustainable society. The Papers are written by members of the Worldwatch Institute research staff and reviewed by experts in the field. Regularly published in five languages, they have been used as concise and authoritative references by governments, nongovernmental organizations, and educational institutions worldwide. For a partial list of available Papers, see back pages.

Table of Contents

ACKNOWLEDGMENTS: We are grateful to Marion Nestle, Barbara MkNelly, John Mason, Mark Ritchie, Francie King, Josefa Eusebio, Clark Larsen, Tim Lang, Ramesh Soman, Lisa Smith, Graham Colditz, and Anne Wolf for sharing expertise, as well as data and information. Barry Popkin, Kelly Brownell, Sonya Rabeneck, Elena McCollim, Rafa Flores, Marc Cohen, Kate Clancy, Ronald Halweil, Susan Horton, and Peter Rosset also provided essential suggestions and criticism on various drafts of the paper.

Thanks to Lester Brown who (almost three decades ago!) conceived of the idea for a Worldwatch paper on the two faces of global malnutrition. Many others at Worldwatch were indispensable in producing this paper. Hilary French, David Roodman, Janet Abramovitz, and Lester Brown reviewed early and late drafts of the paper. Linda Starke edited the *State of the World* chapter that later developed into this paper. And Jane Peterson, the paper editor, revived much of the material pruned from the chapter and helped us to replace jargon with more friendly and understandable language.

Working largely behind the scenes, Liz Doherty transformed text and raw data into the manicured paper you now hold, while Dick Bell, Mary Caron, and Liz Hopper assured that a wide audience would be exposed to our research.

GARY GARDNER is a Senior Researcher at the Worldwatch Institute, where he writes on agriculture, water, and materials use issues. Since joining the Institute in 1994, he has written chapters in the Institute's *State of the World* and *Vital Signs* annuals, and has contributed to *World Watch* magazine. Major research projects include *Shrinking Fields*, which was one of the Institute's contributions to the World Food Summit in Rome in November 1996, and *Recycling Organic Waste*.

BRIAN HALWEIL is a Staff Researcher at the Worldwatch Institute, where he focuses on issues related to food and agriculture, ranging from biotechnology to water scarcity to organic farming. He has contributed to *State of the World* and *Vital Signs*, as well as *World Watch* magazine. Brian also co-authored the book *Beyond Malthus: Nineteen Dimensions of the Population Challenge*.

Introduction

*"Y*ou are what you eat," goes the old adage, a popular way of describing the close links between diet and a person's development. But the diet-development connection also applies to whole societies: *we* are what *we* eat. And this has been true throughout history. Consider, for example, the experience of the Guale people living thousands of years ago near what later became Savannah, Georgia, in the United States.

Daily life for these pre-agricultural people was relatively uncomplicated. Child-rearing, observing religious rituals, and meeting basic needs—especially the gathering of food—filled most of their days. Prehistoric Georgians collected acorns, hickory nuts, walnuts, and persimmons along with other plants, and hunted deer and seafood to meet their daily energy requirements, naturally keeping a balance between what they took in as calories and put out as energy.[1]

As the Guale began to practice agriculture, probably to increase the food supply for a growing population, their diets changed and so did their activities. Now they had plentiful and storable supplies of corn, a grain that previously had been only marginal in their diets, and this agricultural plenty eventually freed many in their tribe to pursue non-farming endeavors such as temple-building and art.[2]

While the shift to agriculture enhanced the lives of the early Georgians in some respects, it also had some negative effects on their diet and health. Diets tied to cultivation of a few major crops lacked the diversity, and therefore the full range of vitamins and minerals, that gatherer-hunters had enjoyed, and made them somewhat less robust. And though episodes of hunger were less frequent, when they did occur they were more severe—often reaching famine levels—than the light bouts of seasonal scarcity experienced by the gatherer-hunters. Moreover, the division of labor made possible by agricultural surpluses soon ossified into a class system in which the quality of one's diet came to reflect one's social standing.[3]

These nutritional and socioeconomic changes worsened the health of the Guale in striking ways. Bones and teeth from their burial sites reveal that the shift to agriculture led to a decrease in body size, bone length, and physical strength. Children, especially those from lower classes, never reached their full potential for growth. Cavities and tooth loss multiplied with the increased consumption of corn, a sugary grain, and with greater use of ceramic pottery, which facilitated food preparation techniques that promoted tooth decay. Finally, the steady food supply encouraged denser settlement, which, in combination with lower dietary quality, provided a fertile environment for outbreaks of tuberculosis and other infectious diseases that had been much less common among gatherer-hunters. By some accounts, even life expectancy fell among the adult population of early agriculturalists.[4]

The story of the early Georgians illustrates the close relationship between diet and development. Major technological and economic innovations, from the Agricultural Revolution beginning 10,000 years ago to the Industrial Revolution starting in the late 18th century, have deeply influenced what and how people eat, with important consequences for their health. While some of these impacts were positive, societies have largely failed to guard against the harm that some innovations in food production, distribution, and preparation have done to the nutrition and health of many people.

In the 20th century, development's impact on nutrition was especially profound. Despite unprecedented wealth and surplus food stocks at the global level, malnutrition spread more widely than at perhaps any time in history. The World Health Organization (WHO) estimates that fully half of the human family, some 3 billion people, suffer from malnutrition of one form or another. Indeed, a survey of U.N.-sponsored studies indicates that hunger afflicts at least 1.2 billion people, while another 1.2 billion consume more than they need, becoming overweight with harmful consequences. Meanwhile, virtually all of the hungry, many of the overweight, and others of normal weight are debilitated by a deficiency of essential vitamins and minerals. (See Table 1.) For all the display of technological and economic prowess in the last century, most countries neglected nutritional well-being, a fundamental building block of societal development. Today, for example, more than half of modern-day Georgian adults are overweight, the result of a pattern of development that has made unhealthy foods and sedentary lifestyles the norm.[5]

The consequences of this epidemic of malnutrition are sobering. Hunger, overeating, and micronutrient deficiencies, for example, account for an estimated half or more of

TABLE 1

Types and Effects of Malnutrition, and Number Affected Globally, 2000

Type of Malnutrition	Nutritional Effect	Number Affected Globally (billion)
Hunger	Deficiency of calories and protein	At least 1.2
Micronutrient Deficiency	Deficiency of vitamins and minerals	2.0–3.5
Overconsumption	Excess of calories often accompanied by deficiency of vitamins and minerals	At least 1.2

Note: Hunger and overconsumption correspond to underweight or overweight populations. There is considerable overlap between micronutrient deficiency and other forms of malnutrition.
Source: See endnote 5.

the world's burden of disease. The harm to individuals and their families, of course, can be devastating: more than 5 million children die of hunger-related diseases each year, while survivors are often physically or mentally stunted, performing well below their potential at school and work. Meanwhile, millions of people in wealthy countries spend years or even decades late in life crippled with heart disease, diabetes, cancer, or other diseases attributable at least in part to overeating. Thus, for both rich and poor, malnutrition means living less than a full life.[6]

Malnutrition also exacts a heavy social toll, slowing and sometimes partly reversing societies' development. Treating the effects of obesity in the United States, for example, costs more than $100 billion annually—more than 10 percent of the nation's bill for healthcare. And hunger destroys would-be Einsteins and Gandhis in childhood, while productivity losses among those who reach adulthood are widespread. A 1999 study of India by the World Bank found that hunger-induced productivity losses cost the economy $10–$28 billion dollars annually, some 3–9 percent of the country's GDP in 1996. Meanwhile, the effects of hunger among women ripple across society: hungry women are less able to provide for their families and to properly nourish their own bodies during pregnancy, which often results in lifelong impairment for their children and a consequent loss of personal and community potential. So whether the problem stems from hunger or from overeating, whether it occurs in poor countries or rich ones, malnutrition is bound to skew and slow a country's development.[7]

While progress has been made in reducing hunger in recent decades, it has often meant simply trading hunger for other forms of malnourishment. Today, overeating and its associated medical costs are spreading rapidly beyond wealthy countries to the developing world. The number of diabetics worldwide whose condition results from overeating is projected to double between 1998 and 2025, with more than three quarters of this growth occurring in the developing world. Unlike wealthy countries, which have largely contained many infectious diseases, developing nations will have to fight a health battle on two fronts, struggling to contain ailments such as heart disease and cancer even as infectious disease continues to afflict masses of people.[8]

The poor record of global nutrition is plainly the result of distorted policy priorities. Where hunger is the problem, policymakers often claim that they lack the resources they need to make headway. But lack of funds is not the main roadblock. Low-income societies such as Cuba and the Indian state of Kerala have substantially reduced or contained hunger, in spite of challenging economic circumstances, simply by making its elimination a policy priority. Kerala, for example, one of the poorest states in India, has a childhood malnutrition rate nearly half that of India as a whole.[9]

Where overeating is the problem, policymakers have typically neglected nutrition education, allowing giant food companies to educate the public and to influence people's food purchases by default through extensive marketing. Food is the most heavily advertised commodity in Austria, France, Belgium, and the United States, and more than half of this advertising is for candy, sweetened breakfast cereals, fast food, and other items of dubious nutritional value. With food companies largely unchallenged in targeting our sweet tooth and shaping our tastes, it is little surprise that more than half of American adults, for example, are overweight and one in five are obese.[10]

For a variety of reasons, the century with the greatest potential to eliminate malnutrition instead saw it boosted to record levels. Still, with increased attention to nutrition and awareness of its impact on health and development, the elimination of hunger and overeating is becoming a realistic policy goal. What is more, the most urgent problems—hunger and lack of essential vitamins and minerals—can often be reversed cheaply, sometimes for as little as a few pennies per person *per year*. Eliminating the root causes of malnutrition—generally poverty in the case of hunger, and a predominance of unhealthy foods and sedentary lifestyles in the case of overeating—is a more challenging task. But a con-

certed effort could yield tremendous benefits for individuals
and nations alike. Once policymakers appreciate the burden
malnutrition places on development, adequate nutrition for
all will become a leading priority.[11]

A Malnourished World

Today our food supply is nothing less than cornucopian,
favoring the world with unprecedented quantities and
varieties of food. Yet more people and a greater proportion of
the world today are malnourished—hungry, deficient in vitamins or minerals, or overfed—than ever before in human
history. To be sure, the three faces of malnutrition are taking
different directions globally. But overall, trends in nutrition,
and trends in the way the food system operates, are headed
down troubling paths. (See Table 2.)[12]

Malnutrition is an imbalance—a deficiency or an
excess—in a person's intake of nutrients and other dietary
elements needed for healthy living. Carbohydrates, protein,
and fat—the macronutrients—provide the basic building
blocks for cellular growth. They are also the body's only
source of energy, or calories: each gram of carbohydrate or
protein provides about four calories; each gram of fat, about
nine. Micronutrients are vitamins and minerals, such as iron,
calcium, and vitamins A through E. They provide no energy
and are consumed in small quantities, but they are essential
nevertheless, helping macronutrients to build and maintain
the body. Cholesterol, fiber, and other components of food
also affect nutrition and health, although they are not
defined as nutrients.[13]

Foods vary widely in their nutrient composition.
Whole grains are mostly carbohydrates, but they also provide
fiber, protein, and small amounts of fat and micronutrients.
Meat's profile is virtually the negative image of grain's, with
large quantities of fat, cholesterol, protein, and some
micronutrients, but no carbohydrates or fiber. Fruits and veg-

TABLE 2

Share of Children Who Are Underweight and Adults Who Are Overweight, Selected Countries, Mid-1990s

Country	Share Underweight (percent)	Country	Share Overweight (percent)
Bangladesh	56	United States	55
India	53	Russian Federation	54
Ethiopia	48	United Kingdom	51
Viet Nam	40	Germany	50
Nigeria	39	Colombia	41
Indonesia	34	Brazil	36

Source: See endnote 12.

etables tend to be low in fat, but rich in fiber and micronutrients. And other foods, such as refined sugar, provide "empty calories"—energy lacking additional nutritional value. Striking a healthy nutrient balance requires eating from each of these categories, but in different quantities. A joint research effort by the Harvard School of Public Health and Oldways Preservation and Exchange Trust found that traditional diets associated with little nutrition-related illness and lengthy adult life expectancies are generally plant-based—rich in whole grains, vegetables, fruits, and nuts—and supplemented by sparing amounts of animal products.[14]

Hunger, the worst of the three forms of malnutrition because it often cuts short lives that have barely begun, has been reduced modestly in recent decades. The U.N. Food and Agriculture Organization (FAO) reports that 790 million people—roughly one out of five people in the developing world—are chronically hungry, down from 918 million in 1970, a drop of 14 percent. This estimate captures the trend but likely underestimates the number of hungry. It is based largely on calculations of calories available per person, a method that does not adequately account for the unequal distribution of food found virtually everywhere. For example, FAO estimates that 21 percent of India's population is chronically undernourished. But recent on-the-ground surveys paint a more accurate and desperate picture: 49 percent of adults and 53 percent of children in India are underweight, a proxy measurement for hunger.[15]

Using underweight among children rather than calories per person as the measuring stick, it becomes apparent that hunger in the developing world has fallen over the past two decades: 26 million fewer children were estimated to be underweight in 2000 than in 1980. (See Table 3.) The greatest absolute progress in reducing hunger was achieved in Asia, while the greatest relative reduction came in Latin America, where the population of underweight children was cut in half. Africa, on the other hand, saw an increase in the number of children who are underweight. There, the number suffering from this condition nearly doubled—spotlighting the continent as an area deserving particular concern.[16]

Despite the progress in some regions, hunger remains stubbornly rooted across much of the developing world. The greatest concentration of chronically hungry people is in

TABLE 3

Underweight Children in Developing Countries, 1980 and 2000

Area	Underweight Children		Share of Children Who Are Underweight	
	1980	2000	1980	2000
	(million)		(percent)	
Africa	22	38	26	29
Asia	146	108	44	29
Latin America and the Caribbean	7	3	14	6
All developing countries	176	150	37	27

Source: See endnote 16.

South Asia and sub-Saharan Africa. Some 44 percent of South Asia's children are underweight, while the shares in India, Bangladesh, and Afghanistan are well above this average. In sub-Saharan Africa, 36 percent of children are underweight, but the figure approaches 50 percent in nations such as Somalia, Ethiopia, and Niger. Even in Latin America, with a relatively small share of hungry people, particular countries and subregions such as Haiti and Central America still have high levels of hunger.[17]

In the developing world, the countryside harbors most of the hungry, the majority of whom are women and children. At the same time, the rapid urbanization that is the dominant trend throughout Latin America, Africa, and Asia means that hunger is becoming increasingly common in major cities. A 1999 study from the International Food Policy Research Institute (IFPRI) found the absolute number and share of undernourished people in urban areas to be on the rise in the majority of developing nations surveyed.[18]

Hunger is found in pockets of the industrial world as well. The U.S. Department of Agriculture (USDA) estimates that in 1998 some 10 percent of U.S. households were "food-insecure"—hungry, on the edge of hunger, or worried about being hungry. These households are home to nearly one in five American children. In Europe, Australia, and Japan, where social safety nets are more widespread, hunger is more rare.[19]

While hunger has receded modestly, its opposite—overeating—is more prevalent today than ever. Indeed, WHO calls the swift spread of the condition of overweight and its extreme form, obesity, "one of the greatest neglected public health problems of our time." Worldwide, the number of overweight people now rivals the number who are underweight. Overweight and obesity are defined using body-mass index (BMI), a scale calibrated to reflect the health effects of weight gain. A healthy BMI ranges from 19 to 24; a BMI of 25 or above indicates "overweight" and brings increased risk of illnesses such as cardiovascular disease, diabetes, and cancer. A BMI above 30 signals "obesity" and even greater health risks.[20]

The United States has spearheaded this overeating wave. Today it is more common than not for American adults to be overweight: 55 percent have a BMI over 25. Moreover, the share of American adults who are obese has climbed from 15 to 23 percent just since 1980. And one out of five American children are now overweight or obese, a 50 percent increase in the last two decades. Meanwhile, the incidence of overweight or obesity in Europe has risen at a similar rate in the last decade, although from somewhat lower levels. The prevalence of obesity in England, for example, has doubled in the last 10 years to 16 percent.[21]

It seems natural to assume that being overweight or obese is strictly a developed-country problem, but this is not true. A 1999 United Nations study found obesity at measurable levels in all developing regions, and growing rapidly, even in countries where hunger persists. In China, for example, the share of adults who are overweight jumped by more than half—from 9 percent to 15 percent—between 1989 and 1992. In several Latin American nations, such as Brazil and Colombia, the prevalence of overweight people—at 36 and 41 percent, respectively—approaches the share in some of Europe. In these and more and more developing countries, it is not uncommon for the overweight population to exceed the underweight population.[22]

The third malnourished population—those with inadequate intakes of vitamins and minerals—partially overlaps with both the hungry and the overfed. Micronutrient deficiencies typically result from a lack of dietary variety—three bowls of rice and little else each day, for example, or frequent consumption of hamburgers and french fries. Low intake of three micronutrients—iodine, vitamin A, and iron—is of particular concern globally because it is so widespread.[23]

The human body needs only one teaspoon of iodine over a lifetime, consumed in tiny amounts. Yet iodine deficiency disorder (IDD), the world's leading preventable cause of mental retardation, affects 740 million people—some 13 percent of the world population—in at least 130 developing countries. (Prevalence of IDD stood at double this level in the mid-1990s, before a worldwide salt-iodization initiative.) Another 2 billion people are reportedly at risk. Vitamin A deficiency (VAD) is less well documented, but data from hard-hit countries in Latin America and Africa indicate that the prevalence ranges from 9 to 50 percent of the population.[24]

The most commonly lacking micronutrient, however, is iron—a mineral found in whole grains, green leafy vegetables, and meat. A 1999 U.N. report estimates that over 70 percent of the developing-world population—3.5 billion people—suffer from varying degrees of iron deficiency. Among the most severely affected, largely women and children in poor countries, lack of iron leads to anemia and cognitive disability.[25]

Changes in hunger, overeating, and micronutrient intake have been linked to changes in eating patterns when traditional diets and food sources are replaced by less nutritious alternatives. On every continent, for instance, the age-old practice of breast-feeding is being replaced by more "modern" alternatives, even though breast milk is the best source of nutrition for infants and protects babies from some illnesses. In only three countries in Latin America is exclusive breast-feeding—the UNICEF recommendation for infants under the age of six months—practiced by more than half of new mothers. And rates are even lower in the industrial world: only 14 percent of mothers in the United States breast-feed exclusively in the first six months.[26]

Today's dinner plates also contain larger servings of fat and sugar than yesterday's did as people eat more and more livestock products and as oil and sweeteners are increasingly added to foods of all kinds. In Europe and North America, fat and sugar account for more than half of caloric intake, and they have squeezed complex carbohydrates, such as grains and vegetables, down to just a third of total calories—a nearly complete reversal of the diet of our gatherer-hunter forebears. Moreover, whole grain products have been largely replaced with refined grains, which are stripped of fiber and of many vitamins and minerals; fully 98 percent of the wheat flour consumed in the United States is refined. And fast-food items, which often surpass government guidelines for daily intake of fat, sugar, cholesterol, and sodium in a single meal, may be displacing nutritious dark green and yellow vegetables: one fifth of the "vegetables" Americans eat are french fries and potato chips. These trends are rapidly spreading beyond industrial nations as the fast-food culture goes global.[27]

Meanwhile, eating in industrial countries centers less and less on home, family, and three square meals. Changes in work and family, food availability and price have made eating a more frequent but less sacred activity. Snacking is commonplace: in 1996, only 24 percent of Americans ate breakfast, lunch, and dinner and nothing else, which is down from 33 percent in 1985. In the United Kingdom, per capita consumption of snack foods, including potato chips, salted nuts, and other savories, is up by nearly a quarter in the past five years; snack foods are now a $3.6 billion industry.[28]

More than ever, meals are eaten out, often on the run: the average American eats one of every three meals outside the home, and one's car is the second most popular place to have breakfast. Given these trends, it is not surprising that Americans cook less than ever. In 1998, just 38 percent of meals eaten in American homes were "homemade"; a recent report from consulting firm McKinsey & Co. suggests that many consumers in 2005 will have never cooked a meal from basic ingredients. In consumption-oriented countries, especially the United States, the nutritional and cultural value of food is increasingly being overwhelmed by its transformation into a money-making product to be grabbed off the shelf.[29]

The Roots of Hunger

Most people would correctly identify hunger as the most critical form of malnourishment. But few can pinpoint its causes. The myth persists today that hunger results from scarce food supplies, and that poor harvests, usually the result of insufficient rainfall or barren soils, are its primary

cause. But in fact hunger is the product of human decisions—especially decisions about how a society is organized.
Whether people have a decent livelihood, what status is
accorded to women, and whether governments are account-
able to their people have far more impact on who eats adequately and who does not than a country's agricultural
endowment does.

Nobel Laureate and economist Amartya Sen argues per-
suasively that poverty—rather than food shortages—is frequently the underlying cause of hunger. Indeed, nearly 80
percent of all malnourished children in the developing world
in the early 1990s lived in countries that boasted food surpluses. The more important feature common to these countries is pervasive poverty, which limits people's access to food
in the market or to land, credit, and other inputs needed to
produce food. Poverty also means poor access to non-food
services, including health care, education, and a clean living
environment, which increases the likelihood of hunger.
Conditions like diarrhea, for instance, usually the result of an
unclean water supply, prevent a child from absorbing available nutrients, while a poor education often means poor job
prospects, with adverse consequences for income, and, in
turn, for nutrition. Recognizing these linkages, the UNICEF
Framework for the Causes of Childhood Malnutrition stress-
es the importance of adequate care for mothers and children
(support for pregnant and lactating mothers and child feeding, play and cognitive stimulation for children) and a proper health environment (safe water, sanitation, and shelter),
both of which are affected by poverty.[30]

Poverty often strikes hardest among women, the nutritional gatekeepers in many families. FAO estimates that more
than half of the world's food is raised by women, and in rural
areas of Africa, Latin America, and Asia, the figure soars to 80
percent. Yet women have little or no access to land ownership, credit, agricultural training, education, and social privileges in general. In five African nations, for example—
Kenya, Malawi, Sierra Leone, Zambia, and Zimbabwe—at
least 40 percent of the people are chronically hungry, and

women do most of the farming, yet women receive less than 10 percent of the credit awarded to smallholders and just 1 percent of agricultural credit overall, which limits their ability to increase income and boost nutrition.[31]

Women in developing countries reinvest nearly all of their earned income to meet household food and other needs, whereas men often set aside up to a quarter of their income for alcohol, sex, and other nonhousehold expenses. But women impoverished to the point of hunger bear hungry children, and are less able to care for their offspring and to breast-feed, and these conditions perpetuate hunger across generations. In sum, societies that abandon women to poverty are weakening one of their key defenses against malnutrition.[32]

Poverty and hunger can also result from a range of well-intentioned policies when leaders fail to consider their specific impact on the poor and hungry. The Green Revolution of the 1960s and 1970s is a case where policy benefits were undermined as a result of this failure. Researchers focused on boosting the yields of a narrow base of cereals—primarily corn, wheat, and rice—which led to a huge increase in caloric availability, a nutritional plus. But gains in cereal production often came at the expense of cultivation of more nutritious legumes, root crops, and other grains. The growing dominance of cereals resulted in reduced dietary diversity, which has contributed to widespread micronutrient deficiencies. In South Asia, for example, per capita grain consumption increased 13 percent in the last 40 years, but per capita consumption of legumes—which are higher in protein and many vitamins and minerals—has dropped more than 50 percent.[33]

Meanwhile, the Green Revolution's emphasis on purchased fertilizer and pesticides and on irrigated cultivation tended to favor those with easy access to financing and agricultural infrastructure. Larger, wealthier farmers—rather than those desperate to improve their productivity and incomes—were first to adopt these costly yield-enhancing technologies, in some cases exacerbating existing inequalities in land holdings and income. This bias toward privileged farmers perpetuates long-standing government policies in many nations. In Mexico, for example, between 1940 and 1970, some 60 percent of all government investment in agriculture went to the large irrigated farms of Sinaloa and Sonora—where only 9 percent of Mexico's farmers are located. A different Green Revolution, one focused on increasing output of a variety of crops and directed at small farmers, would likely have left a greater nutritional legacy than the one that actually took place.[34]

Where governments have allowed land to be concentrated in a few hands, rural poverty and hunger tend to be most severe—especially in situations where land ownership is required to obtain credit or other assistance. In India, where 5 percent of the farm households control nearly 60 percent of the land, landless people are considerably more likely to be malnourished than other rural inhabitants.[35]

Another common policy whose implementation has not always been sensitive to the needs of the poor is structural adjustment. Structural adjustment programs (SAPs), which are frequently pushed by international lending organizations such as the International Monetary Fund (IMF) and the World Bank, are intended to help nations revive their economies and service international debts, typically by slashing public spending and promoting export industries. These programs are often biased against the poor and can erode nutritional conditions, especially when governments opt to protect military budgets and corporate welfare at the expense of food subsidies, agricultural credit, health and education expenditures, and other public services critical to nutritionally vulnerable populations. One of the most comprehensive assessments of the effects of adjustment on human welfare, the UNICEF-sponsored *Adjustment with a Human Face*, documented increases in stunting, underweight, and low birth weight in the wake of structural adjustment policies in nine of 11 Latin American, African, and Asian nations surveyed in the 1980s. Although the IMF and the World Bank refer increasingly to the need for social safety nets, recent assessments of the impact of SAPs on nutrition indicate that implementation of this idea on the ground is still inadequate.[36]

In order to earn foreign exchange that can pay down their loans, many indebted countries promote the export of coffee, bananas, flowers, and other cash crops. Without an effort by government to ensure that small farmers get a piece of the export pie, large corporations, foreign investors, and large landowners are typically the chief beneficiaries of such an orientation. An assessment of the surge in nontraditional agricultural exports—such as baby broccoli or cut flowers—in Chile, Paraguay, and Guatemala found "a significant loss of land over time by small and middle-sized producers, and the concentration of land in the hands of large growers." Because larger farms tend to be less labor intensive, at least in the short term, this transformation meant a net decrease in rural employment, with negative effects on rural income and nutrition.[37]

The growing emphasis on free trade in agricultural products brings additional nutritional vulnerabilities. Current trade arrangements, such as the Agreement on Agriculture under the World Trade Organization (WTO), permit the industrial farmers of Europe and North America to sell subsidized grain, oils, and other commodity surpluses cheaply in developing nations, undercutting local farmers and forcing many off the land—their source of nutrition security. In most cases, any benefits of this cheap food to the urban poor are likely to be transitory, as the destabilization of the rural economy encourages migration to job-scarce cities, thereby increasing the ranks of impoverished city dwellers while harming urban agriculture programs.[38]

Meanwhile, dependence on foreign markets for staple foods leaves importing countries vulnerable to price fluctuations and currency devaluations that can increase the price of food substantially. Mexican consumers, for example, initially benefited from cheap imports of corn from the United States under the North American Free Trade Agreement (NAFTA). But when the peso was devalued in 1995, the price of imported corn doubled in one year, making corn more expensive

throughout the domestic market. Some hungry Mexicans—
including farmers undercut by the flood of American corn—
took to looting rail freight cars to obtain food.[39]

While hunger can spark social unrest, the reverse is also
true: conflict can often produce or worsen hunger. From
Angola to Kosovo, millions are hungry because warring fac-
tions use food as a weapon, choking distribution channels or
forcing people from their farmland. War can exacerbate
hunger by destroying crops, eliminating jobs, and driving up
food prices. And the destruction of agricultural infrastructure, schools, hospitals, and factories means that war's damage to nutrition persists long after the conflict has ended. In
Afghanistan, landmines planted in conflicts since 1979 prevent an estimated half to two thirds of the nation's arable
land from being tilled. A rash of civil wars and resulting
refugee flows in central Africa in the 1990s are at the center
of the worsening hunger there.[40]

The Nutrition Transition

While prosperity this last century bypassed millions, it
swept millions more to new diets that were often
bountiful, but nutritionally deficient. Traditional diets fea-
turing grains and vegetables gave way to foods heavy in fat
and sugar, even as a shift to sedentary work and leisure activities demanded fewer calories. The new dietary patterns,
however, did not emerge spontaneously from farms and
kitchens worldwide. Instead, this "nutrition transition" was
part of a series of interrelated transitions—in economics,
demographics, and health—that together helped to define
industrial development in the 20th century.

Just as the transition from hunting and gathering to agriculture millennia ago helped create social inequality, the transitions underlying 20th century development also skewed
society in various ways. Economic growth was often accompanied by an increase in income inequality, for example, and

disease patterns affected rich and poor differently. These skewings affected nutrition, usually for the worse, while poor nutrition, in turn, looped back to exacerbate most of these inequalities. (See Table 4.)[41]

The story of dietary change begins not with these development threads but with humanity's innate love of sweets and fats. These preferences were crucial for enabling people to store energy and weather lean times in hunter-gatherer days when energy-dense foods were scarce. Compounding this preference is the fact that sugary and fatty foods are easy to overconsume because the human body has weak satiation mechanisms for fat and sugar. By contrast, foods high in fiber and complex carbohydrates, such as whole grain bread and potatoes, leave us feeling full. Despite a craving for the calorie-charged foods, earlier societies consumed them in relatively small quantities simply because they were not extensively available.[42]

Availability of food in general increased, of course, as economic and technological innovations revolutionized agriculture and society. Mechanization of farming, widespread use of fertilizer and irrigation, and the breeding of high-yielding crops all served to boost the supply of foods in wealthy and poor nations alike. And improvements in transportation, packaging, and marketing helped to distribute this cornucopian supply broadly. The increased availability of meat, milk, cheese, sugar, and other sweet and fatty foods—commodities once reserved for the affluent or for holidays—was instrumental in facilitating a transition to a richer diet.[43]

At the same time, industrialization created wealth at levels never seen before, giving more people the means to adopt the new diet. Consider the case of China, where per capita income grew fourfold after the economic reforms of 1978. Consumption of high-fat foods such as pork and soy oil (which is used for frying) both soared, while consumption of rice and starchy roots dropped. The Chinese experience illustrates the trend found nearly everywhere: when impoverished people experience a bit of prosperity, one of

TABLE 4

Changes in Four Societal Sectors during the Transition from Preindustrial to Industrial Society

Sector Affected	Advances in Each Sector	Skewing
Economy	Agricultural modernization increases the food supply and industrialization raises national income.	But income and food distribution is highly unequal in the transition from preindustrial to industrial society.
Population	Advances in nutrition and health reduce death rates.	But birth rates remain high, leading to a demographic imbalance that fuels population growth. Eventually, birth rates fall into line with death rates, but not among the poor, who continue to see high rates of birth.
Diet	Food supply becomes abundant, diverse, and more affordable.	But the poor remain undernourished, while the wealthy eat too many foods with little nutritional value. Eventually, fat and sugar become cheaper, and obesity increases among the poor as well.
Health	Infectious disease recedes.	But "diseases of affluence" emerge among the prosperous as diets and lifestyles change. Meanwhile, the poor continue to suffer from infectious disease. Eventually, the poor suffer from diseases of affluence as well, as nutritionally poor foods become more affordable.

Source: See endnote 41.

their highest priorities is to broaden their diet, typically by consuming greater quantities of foods high in fat, such as cooking oil and livestock products.[44]

Of course, increases in income are not spread evenly across most societies, and skewed incomes typically lead to a skewing of diets by social class. In China between 1989 and 1993, the share of wealthy households consuming a low-fat diet (less than 10 percent of calories from fat) dropped from 11 percent to 2 percent, and the percentage consuming a high-fat diet (more than 30 percent of calories from fat) jumped from 23 percent to 67 percent. For countries undergoing the nutrition transition, a skewing of incomes often leads to a skewing of nutritional patterns, with hunger and overweight found simultaneously in a national population. This skewing is sometimes found even within households, possibly because of gender and generational biases. In China, Russia, and Brazil, for example, 25 to 57 percent of households with an undernourished family member also have a family member who is overweight.[45]

Not only did masses of people prosper this last century, but the level of wealth needed to shift to a fatty diet has fallen in recent decades. In 1962, a diet whose share of calories from fat was 20 percent correlated with a GNP per person of $1,475. By 1990 the same diet correlated with a per capita GNP of only $750 (both figures are 1992 dollars). The reason for this dramatic change is that increased agricultural productivity and new forms of food processing have boosted the availability of cheap fats, especially vegetable oils and meat and animal products. The surge in global vegetable oil production over the past four decades, for example, has added 30 grams of fat to the average diet on the planet. (See Figure 1). In sum, hundreds of millions of low-income people indulge in a richer diet today than was possible several decades ago, and as the Chinese case demonstrates, their shift to a fatty diet can come about faster. Nutrition changes that occurred over the course of half a century in Japan took root in the Chinese diet in just two decades—at much lower income levels.[46]

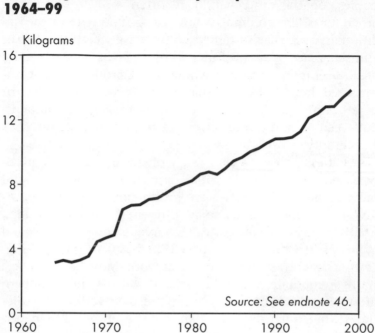

FIGURE 1

World Vegetable Oil Consumption per Person, 1964–99

Kilograms

Source: See endnote 46.

Meanwhile, the surge in agricultural productivity and in prosperity helped to fuel a key demographic trend this century—migration to cities—which had profound consequences for nutrition. With the mechanization of agriculture and the rise of industry, workers once needed on farms were now in demand in urban areas. This change in labor patterns, along with the hope of increased income and a more stimulating life in cities, prompted a mass migration that lifted the urban share of global population from just 10 percent in 1900 to nearly 50 percent today. The new homes, jobs, and lifestyles in urban areas also meant new diets, for a host of disparate reasons.[47]

Cities offer a greater range of food choices, generally at lower prices, than are found in rural areas, at least in poorer nations. A recent study of 133 developing countries found that migration to the city—without any changes in income—can more than double per capita intake of sweeteners, simply because they are cheaply available. Traditional staples, on the other hand, are often more expensive in urban areas. The common result is a shift away from the traditional foods that sustained countless generations. Urban Tunisians, for example, increasingly favor refined white bread over more-nutritious whole wheat products. And cash-squeezed households in Guayaquil, Ecuador, often spurn potatoes and fresh fruit juices in favor of fried plantains, potato chips, and soft drinks, replacing nutrient-dense foods with empty calories.[48]

Cities also offer a wide range of stimuli that are typically absent in the countryside. Exposure to television and movies, many of them western productions that feature carnivorous dietary habits, may influence dietary attitudes. Analysis from the China Health Survey shows that demand for meat in China has outpaced increases in income, suggesting that other influences are at work. Meat has become a status symbol in China, associated with a more modern lifestyle and a move away from the deprivation of earlier times when a largely vegetarian diet was enforced by poverty, not choice.[49]

Migration to cities also means changing roles for women, which in turn can affect nutrition. Many women begin to work outside the home after moving to cities, and have little time to purchase, prepare, serve, and clean up food, a situation worsened by the common failure of men to shoulder their share of these chores. Time pressures also dissuade many women from breast-feeding. These social changes make prepared and processed foods—which are often high in fat, cholesterol, and sugar and low in fiber, vitamins, and minerals—increasingly attractive. Indeed, the rapid rise in female labor and dual-income families following World War II is commonly linked to the popularity of convenience foods in industrial countries, a trend that continues to unfold in developing countries today.[50]

Even as more calories become available to city dwellers, fewer are needed for daily living. Urban work tends to demand less physical exertion than farm work did. As the share of developing-country populations engaged in agriculture has declined from roughly 80 percent in 1950 to 55 percent today, more people earn their living in jobs with limited physical challenges. Meanwhile, at home, physically demanding food preparation techniques, such as the grinding of grains, kneading of dough, and pounding of roots are often replaced in cities by machines or by prepared foods and ingredients. And electrified labor-saving amenities at home, motorized transportation, and sedentary leisure activities further lower energy expenditure.[51]

Migration to the city can more than double per capita intake of sweeteners.

Despite the reduced need for calories, many people maintain high-calorie diets in cities, increasing the incidence of overweight and a shift in disease patterns that parallels the transitions in economics, demographics, and nutrition. Some 23 percent of Chinese urbanites are overweight, for example, compared with just over 10 percent of rural Chinese. The new urban patterns of eating, combined with a sedentary lifestyle lead to a surge in cardiovascular illness, diabetes, cancer, and other noncommunicable conditions that once afflicted only emperors and kings. This shift in disease patterns is especially challenging for developing nations, which must cope with a sudden rise in chronic disease before they have tamed infectious diseases.[52]

, On the other hand, a budding nutritional trend offers some hope that choosing between care for the rich and care for the poor can be minimized. Growing awareness of the ills of the industrial diet is prompting elites in the United States, Brazil, Thailand, and Chile, for example, to spurn junk foods, improve exercise habits, and embrace nutritional basics—a diet low in fat and added sugar and high in whole grains, fruits, and vegetables. This countertrend—perhaps the first wave of a new nutrition transition—is inverting the traditional skewed relationship between obesity and socioeconomic levels: the wealthiest often have the best eating habits and maintain proper weight, while the poorest, with little access to healthy food and nutrition education, are increasingly likely to be overweight. In the United States, lower-income Hispanic and African American populations have obesity rates 50 percent higher than those of white populations. The question is whether better eating will spread from elites to entire societies, or whether obesity will become a poor person's disease worldwide. The answer will depend on—and heavily influence—the direction of a country's development.[53]

Promoting Overeating

While urbanization, prosperity, and other social forces paved the way to poor diets for many in the 20th century, it was action—and sometimes, inaction—by consumers, food companies, and governments that led to overeating and the consumption of empty calories. None of these groups set out to sabotage public health, of course. But with no one acting as a nutritional watchdog, the overwhelming strength of the food industry and the relative passivity of governments left consumers vulnerable to overeating and poor diet.

The strength of the food industry emerges from the same social trends that produced the nutrition transition. While urban migration stretched, weakened, and eventually snapped the connection between farmer and consumer, and while changing lifestyles and rising incomes encouraged more convenience in foods, the food industry stepped in to meet consumer demand—and to shape it. As processors and packagers, and especially as promoters of food, corporations grew in their capacity to create a food environment that makes unhealthy food ubiquitous in modern life.

Food companies' most powerful tool for shaping this environment is advertising. In Austria, Belgium, France, and the United States, food companies spend more on advertising—an estimated $30 billion annually in the United States—than any other industry. Food ad expenditures in the developing world are lower, but they are growing fast as incomes rapidly increase. In Southeast Asia, for example, food ad expenditures tripled between 1984 and 1990, from $2 billion to $6 billion.[54]

Such heavy spending would not be sustained, of course, unless it were having an impact. Sales and marketing figures are often protected information, which makes a direct connection between ad spending and sales difficult to establish. But even U.S.-government-funded promotion campaigns— which are considerably less flashy than most private advertising efforts—have shown a clear relationship between ad expenditure and increased sales of milk, cheese, pork, and orange juice. And in the 1970s, the aggressive marketing of infant formula accounted at least in part for the reduced incidence and duration of breast-feeding worldwide.[55]

The most heavily advertised foods tend to be of dubious nutritional value. A 1996 Consumers International study found that candy, sweetened breakfast cereals, and fast-food restaurants accounted for over half of all food ads in Norway, Australia, the United States, and 10 European Union nations. In the United States, fast-food restaurants alone account for one third of food advertising expenditures. And among all companies—not just food companies— Coca-Cola and McDonald's are among the top 10 advertisers worldwide.[56]

Canny food advertisers disproportionately target children, the least savvy consumers, confident that early influences shape lifelong habits. Studies indicate that food ads boost children's consumption of heavily advertised foods, prompt children to request these foods from caretakers, and stimulate purchases by the children themselves. In a recent study of fourth- and fifth-grade students, heavy viewing of television—the dominant ad delivery mechanism for kids— was a strong predictor of poor nutritional habits, including frequent snacking, and heavy viewers were more likely to believe that fast food was as nutritious as a meal prepared at home. While a sweet tooth is a natural human characteristic, other studies establish that repeated exposure to sweet and fatty foods in childhood sets up a craving for these unhealthy items that is extremely difficult to resist.[57]

In theory, companies could promote nutritious foods, such as apples and carrots, instead of potato chips and cookies. But two factors compel advertisers to focus on sweet and fatty foods. First, they know that consumers will always have a special interest in these products, given an innate preference for them. Second, processed foods are most likely to have "added value"—the alterations or packaging that allow a company to earn higher profits. Doughnuts, for example, will fetch a greater profit than the flour, oil, eggs, and sugar in them would if sold separately. Part of the profit is reinvested in advertising the product, which keeps the cycle of promotion and sales in constant motion. The disproportionate advertising attention on nutritionally bankrupt foods reinforces demand for such foods in a self-perpetuating cycle that neither seller nor buyer can easily break. John Connor, a food economist at Purdue University, notes that "once a company has created a high margin product with a stable market, the revenues are generally sunk into further advertising to keep the market share high and boost consumption of that category of products."[58]

Not all processed foods are nutritionally poor, of course. But when, as often happens, the added "value" is sugar, salt, fats, or oils, the result is usually a tasty and profitable product that is irresistible to consumers and companies alike. Sugar and salt are the two ingredients most widely added to food, and fats and oils are also added in large doses. Consumers are often unaware of the quantities of these additives they are eating, especially where nutritional labeling is not present or is unclear. In 1909, when processed foods were much less common, two thirds of discretionary sugar consumed in the United States was added in the household. Today, three quarters is added during the processing of food, out of the consumer's sight. No wonder Americans consume

70 kilograms of caloric sweeteners per year, nearly 200 grams, or 53 teaspoonfuls, each day. That's seventy-five percent more than in 1909.[59]

Value added generates the revenues needed to fund other marketing strategies in addition to advertising, including product placement, distribution, and efforts to expand the reach of junk food. In the United States, for instance, it is estimated that food manufacturers spend roughly twice as much on promotions aimed at retailers and wholesalers as they do on promotions to consumers, hoping to win prime locations on increasingly crowded supermarket shelves or to figure prominently in supermarket ads. The latest variation on such strategies is Pepsico's "Power of One" campaign, which involves devoting entire aisles of supermarkets exclusively to Pepsi's snack foods and sodas. In preliminary trials, sales of Frito-Lay potato chips, a Pepsi-owned brand, rose 21 percent, while sales of soft drinks—all kinds, not just Pepsi's—increased by 10 percent. Indeed, this strategy boosts not only Pepsi sales, but sales across the category of snack foods.[60]

Americans consume nearly 200 grams, or 53 teaspoonfuls, of caloric sweeteners each day.

The marketing prowess of fast-food firms makes them a growing presence even in areas traditionally free of commercial interest, such as schools. More than 5,000 U.S. schools—13 percent of the country's total—have contracts with fast-food establishments to provide either food service, vending machines, or both. Since 1990, soda companies have offered millions of dollars to cash-strapped school districts in the United States for exclusive rights to sell their products in the schools. Sometimes these lucrative deals require schools to guarantee a minimum level of sales—a clause that prompted School District 11 in Colorado Springs to move vending machines to high-traffic areas and to push Coca-Cola consumption, even in classrooms, when sales fell below expectations in 1998.[61]

Among the newest marketing strategies is the "supersizing" of french fries, popcorn, pizzas, soda, and other fast-food items—at little extra cost to the consumer. The standard 6.5-ounce soda container of the 1950s, for example, has been supplanted by 20-ounce bottles, and one U.S. convenience store pushes a 64-ounce, 600-calorie "Double Gulp" soda bucket. The extra food content costs manufacturers little, since the ingredients account for a tiny share of the sale price; the consumer is paying mostly for the brand name, packaging, and marketing. To the consumer, such a "good value" is highly enticing. But supersizing may be skewing peoples' conception of what a "normal" serving is: in 1998, surveyed Americans consistently labeled as "medium" portions that were double or triple the size of USDA's "medium" guidelines. And consumer behavior studies show that people consistently consume more when they eat from larger containers.[62]

Corporate influence on dietary choice works through more subtle means as well. In the United States, food lobbyists have long pressured federal agencies to soften dietary guidelines that may dampen sales. For example, since 1977, under pressure from meat producers, federal dietary norms changed from "decrease consumption of meat" to "have two or three (daily) servings" and, most recently, to "choose lean meat." And the Dairy Council, which represents the dairy industry, remains the primary provider of nutrition education to elementary school students in the United States—supplying half of all schools with textbooks and other materials.[63]

On the international front, the Codex Alimentarius Commission, the international body that advises the WTO on food standards—including issues related to nutritional labeling, food safety, and additives—is under heavy corporate influence. Research conducted during the 1991 to 1993 cycle of Codex meetings found that of all the non-governmental participants, a full 96 percent represented industry. The 662 representatives from industry easily outweighed the 26 participants from nutrition, public health, or other public interest groups. Despite subsequent calls for Codex reform, recent analysis shows that little has changed. At the

1997 Codex food-labeling committee, for instance, the U.S. delegation consisted of eight government officials, 10 industry executives, and three representatives of nongovernmental organizations (NGOs).[64]

Whatever the corporate strategy, in most nations advertising and other forms of industry influence dwarf government efforts at nutrition education. In the United States, the 3 billion dollars of advertising by fast-food restaurants and the billions more spent promoting snack foods, soda, candy, and sugary breakfast cereals makes USDA's $333 million budget for nutrition education look like a pittance. Kellogg's spends $40 million to promote Frosted Flakes alone. This imbalance in information and power between industry, consumers, and government results in what Kelly Brownell, a Yale University psychologist, has labeled a "toxic food environment": unprecedented access to high-calorie foods that are low in cost, heavily promoted, and good-tasting. Food sellers, of course, see such ubiquity as cause for celebration. In a recent annual report, the Coca-Cola Company described its goal to "make Coca-Cola the preferred drink for any occasion," by putting its products "within reach, wherever you look: at the supermarket, the video store, the soccer field, the gas station—everywhere."[65]

As these strategies run their course in increasingly saturated industrial markets, and as incomes rise in developing nations, many food companies are looking overseas for greater profits. Mexico recently surpassed the United States as the top per capita consumer of Coca-Cola, for example. And that company's 1998 annual report marvels at Africa's rapid population growth and low per capita consumption of carbonated beverages, noting that "Africa represents a land of opportunity for us." The number of American fast-food restaurants overseas is growing rapidly: four of the five new restaurants that McDonald's opens every day are found outside the United States. Facilitated by trade liberalization and the streamlining of investment regulations, foreign direct investment at all levels of the food industry—the primary means by which food corporations boost sales in overseas

markets—is soaring. From Caracas to Calcutta, the same
foods that are jeopardizing health in the industrial world are
now tempting urbanites in the developing world.[66]

How Diet Shapes Health

Hunger, deficiencies of micronutrients, and overeating
are all closely linked to health, suppressing or promoting diseases from the common cold to cancer. Sometimes
diet's influence on disease is direct, as with the capacity of
iodine deficiency to cause mental retardation. Other times
diet interacts with lifestyle patterns to set off a chain reac-
tion: increased fat and sugar consumption, for example,
combined with more sedentary activities typically leads to
obesity, which raises the risk of developing heart disease, diabetes, and hypertension. Whatever the path, researchers are
increasingly confident that a large share of many diseases
can be blamed on poor nutrition. (See Table 5.)[67]

In some ways, the undernourished and overnourished
run similar health risks: both are more susceptible to disease
and both have reduced life expectancies. But important dif-
ferences exist as well. Hunger and the lack of vitamins and
minerals do their greatest damage early in life, while overeating degrades the body gradually, with heart disease, cancer,
and other chronic ailments striking typically in middle and
old age. Moreover, the effects of undernourishment, such as
stunted growth and blindness, are often irreversible, while
illnesses from overeating can often be tamed through
changes in diet and lifestyle.

An assessment of worldwide disease undertaken early
in the 1990s by the World Bank and Harvard University cap-
tured the broad impact of malnutrition on health. The study
measured "years of healthy life lost" because of death or
disability resulting from various risk factors. Hunger and
micronutrient deficiencies are now regarded as the top
two causes for loss of a year of healthy life: updated analysis

TABLE 5

Health Problems That Could Be Avoided through Dietary Change

Disease or Condition	Share of Cases Preventable through a Change in Diet (percent)	Public Initiatives That Could Lower the Risk of Disease or Condition
Cancer	30–40	Promote the consumption of fruits and vegetables; promote low-fat diets and higher levels of physical activity.
Coronary Heart Disease	17–22	Promote low-fat diets and higher levels of physical activity.
Childhood Blindness	over 95	Establish vitamin A supplementation programs; promote consumption of vegetables.
Mental Retardation	33–43	Iodize salt.
Adult-Onset Diabetes	24–66	Promote low-fat diets and higher levels of physical activity.

Source: See endnote 67.

by Dr. John Mason, who worked on the original study, finds hunger to be responsible globally for 22 percent of these losses, and micronutrient deficiencies for 18 percent. The study did not measure the contribution of being overweight, but Dr. Alan Lopez, head of the Harvard study team, is confident that overeating is responsible for at least as large a share of global illness as hunger. Thus, even considering some overlap between micronutrient deficiencies and the two other forms of malnutrition, poor nutrition would easily account for more than half of the global burden of disease.[68]

Some of hunger's worst effects are sown even before a child is born. A 1999 U.N. report on nutrition estimates that each year some 17 million infants—16 percent of all live births—are underweight in the womb, the result of malnutrition in the mother. These children are scarred for life, suffering from impaired immune systems, neurological damage, and retarded physical growth. Underweight *in utero* translates in adulthood to a reduction of five centimeters in height and five kilos in weight.[69]

The consequences of malnutrition in the womb may be broader, however. Epidemiologist David Barker of the University of Southampton hypothesizes—and many nutritionists agree—that *in utero* malnutrition may predispose a person to chronic disease in later life. Barker's theory is that malnutrition in a fetus triggers metabolic and physiologic responses that help it to survive hunger. The same adaptive responses later in life, when food is more plentiful, can lead to high blood pressure, cardiovascular disease, and glucose intolerance, a risk factor for diabetes. The terrible irony of Barker's hypothesis is that a child born hungry might escape the "diseases of poverty" only to be at increased risk of dying from a "disease of affluence."[70]

Many underweight infants, however, do not survive to see adulthood. The risk of death for an infant born at two thirds of normal weight is 10 times greater than for a normal-weight baby. Barker observes that 60 percent of all newborns in India would be in intensive care had they been born in California. And WHO estimates that of the five leading causes of child death in the developing world, 54 percent of cases have malnutrition as an underlying condition.[71]

Hungry infants—and older children and adults as well—are also more susceptible to infectious disease because they lack the energy needed to fight such illness. Infectious disease, in turn, often prevents a hungry body from absorbing the few nutrients it does get. Diarrhea, for example, sweeps away nutrients before they are used. Thus hunger and sickness chase each other in a vicious circle known as the malnutrition-infection cycle.[72]

Even if a person gets sufficient calories, micronutrient deficiencies can take a heavy toll on development and health. Iodine deficiency, as noted earlier, can stunt physical and mental growth, leading to mental retardation in severe cases. And vitamin A deficiency is the world's leading cause of preventable blindness. It is also a killer—researchers have learned that eliminating VAD can reduce infant mortality by an average of 25 percent. Meanwhile, iron deficiency is a particular concern for women because of blood loss during menstruation: some 44 percent of all women in developing countries, and 56 percent of pregnant women there, suffer from anemia, compared with 33 percent of men. Most micronutrient deficiencies in expectant mothers will damage the unborn child. Severe anemia, for example, is a major cause of mental impairment *in utero*.[73]

The nutrition transition essentially trades diseases of dietary deficiency for diseases of dietary excess.

Some micronutrient deficiencies are widespread in industrial nations as well, especially among poorer people. As calorie-rich junk foods push healthy items from the diet, obesity often masks nutrient starvation. In the United States, iron deficiency affects nearly 20 percent of all premenopausal women—and 42 percent of all poor, pregnant African-American women. And the excesses of industrial-nation diets also adversely affect micronutrient levels: extremely high protein intake—characteristic of diets dominated by animal products—tends to leach calcium from bones, heightening the risk of osteoporosis.[74]

As a country grows wealthier, and as people begin to overconsume calories and to eat nutrition-poor foods, a major shift occurs in health patterns. Hospitals see fewer cases of infectious disease and more cases involving chronic illness, including obesity, cardiovascular disease, diabetes, and cancer. The nutrition transition, in other words, spawns an epidemiological transition—essentially trading diseases of dietary deficiency for diseases of dietary excess.[75]

Two long-term surveys have helped establish the link between dietary habits and the prevalence of chronic disease. The China Health Survey has tracked 6,500 Chinese undergoing the nutrition transition since 1983, and found strong correlations between high intake of fat and protein, particularly from animal sources, and the incidence of heart disease, stroke, and colorectal and breast cancer. Meanwhile, the Framingham Heart Study tracked more than 5,000 residents of Framingham, Massachusetts, since the 1950s and found that chronic illness is not a normal or inevitable consequence of aging but is closely tied to modifiable dietary and exercise habits. The long-term nature of these studies, and their broad coverage, make them reliable chronicles of the effect of poor eating on health.[76]

Diets high in calories and fat encourage obesity, which raises the risk of heart disease, stroke, diabetes, and various cancers. These four sets of disease are responsible for more than half of all deaths in the industrial world. High-calorie, high-fat diets also promote high blood pressure and clogged arteries, which are additional risk factors for a variety of degenerative diseases. Dr. Graham Colditz at the Harvard School of Public Health has estimated that among obese American adults, slimming to a healthy weight and maintaining it could prevent 96 percent of diabetes cases, 74 percent of hypertension, 72 percent of coronary heart disease, 32 percent of colon cancers, and 23 percent of breast cancers. Indeed, researchers at the World Cancer Research Fund and the American Institute for Cancer Research (WCRF/AICR) report that changes in diet alone could prevent 30–40 percent of all cancers worldwide—at least as many cases as could be prevented by a cessation of smoking, a more familiar cause of cancer.[77]

People who are overweight also suffer disproportionately from a range of nonlethal but debilitating conditions, including osteoarthritis, hormonal disorders, asthma, sleep apnea, back pain, and infertility. And like underweight, obesity raises the susceptibility to infection by impairing immune function.[78]

The most dramatic health effect of the surge in global

obesity is the parallel rise in diabetes. The global population with adult-onset diabetes jumped nearly fivefold between 1985 and 1998, from 30 million to an estimated 143 million. And the age range of the affected population is broadening rapidly as well. Adult-onset diabetes—the type that is usually associated with being overweight—was once rare in people under 40. But up to 20 percent of new pediatric patients at Columbia University's Naomi Berrie Diabetes Center had adult-onset diabetes in 1998, compared with less than 4 percent in the early 1990s—a trend confirmed at clinics around the United States. As obesity spreads to younger populations, it is likely that other "adult" diseases—from heart disease to stroke and cancer—will also strike young people more frequently.[79]

This growing wave of chronic disease will hit developing countries hardest in the coming decades. The International Diabetes Federation estimates that the number of diabetics worldwide will double to 300 million by 2025, with three quarters of the growth coming in developing nations. And the share of deaths from cancer is projected to double in developing countries to 14 percent by 2015, while holding steady in industrial countries at 18 percent. Of even greater concern is recent epidemiological evidence that non-Caucasian populations, particularly Pacific Islanders, American Indians, Asian Indians, and Mesoamericans and other Hispanics, appear to be susceptible to some chronic diseases, especially adult-onset diabetes, at lower levels of overweight and at younger ages than Caucasians.[80]

Societal Costs of Poor Diet

The toll of malnutrition on society is broader but perhaps more subtle than its impact on individual health. Children's performance at school, worker productivity, the size of the national health budget—all of these are affected by malnutrition. Most studies of this effect are partial, analyzing hunger but not obesity, for example, or the impact on children but not adults. But they suggest a huge cost to society and yield a clear conclusion: malnutrition hampers a country's development—in poor nations, by making them less productive and less prosperous; in wealthy nations, by paring back hard-won development gains such as lower levels of disability and longer life spans.

Nutritional deficiencies often hamper children's capacity to learn. The World Bank reports that undernutrition and micronutrient deficiencies together result in a 5 to 10 percent loss in learning capacity. And a set of nine studies on nutrition's role in educational performance suggests that early malnutrition can affect school aptitudes, concentration, and attentiveness and can lead to delays in starting school. In Spain and Indonesia, children in areas with high levels of iodine deficiency reportedly average three fewer years in school than their peers in comparable but nondeficient communities. In the Philippines, a 12-year study of more than 2,000 children linked stunting during infancy to a marked increase in the dropout rate, later enrollment in school, and poorer school performance.[81]

Meanwhile, hunger among adults reduces their strength and physical stamina, which lowers productivity at work. For five South Asian nations, economist Susan Horton of the University of Toronto estimates that productivity losses range from 2 to 6 percent for adults who were moderately malnourished and stunted in childhood, and from 2 to 9 percent for those who were severely malnourished. Fatigue induced by iron deficiency is especially devastating: for light blue-collar work, productivity losses are measured at 5 percent, and for heavy manual labor, at 17 percent.[82]

Horton also expressed these productivity reductions in terms of lost wages. She calculates that productivity losses from hunger and micronutrient deficiencies cost South Asian countries 1–2 percent of their gross domestic product each year in lost wages. A modest-sounding sum, these losses nevertheless amount to more than $5 billion annually for these five countries together—equal to their total government health budgets. Horton's pathbreaking work is conservative: it does not measure the costs associated with child deaths, premature births, disruption to the immune system, the cognitive effects related to stunting, and less quantifiable consequences of undernutrition. And her analysis is consistent with more recent and broader studies on the toll of malnutrition: the World Bank estimated in 1999 that malnutrition costs India $10–28 billion in lost productivity, illness, and death each year. This total represents 3 to 9 percent of the country's 1996 GDP, and is greater than its budget for nutrition, health, and education combined.[83]

Malnutrition takes a great toll on productivity in industrial countries as well. In a 1994 study of 80,000 Americans, obese participants were found to account for a disproportionate share of health-related absences from work. For example, they were half again as likely as other study participants to take sick days in bed. And a 1995 study from Sweden estimated that obesity accounted for 7 percent of lost productivity due to sick leave and disability, and that the obese were twice as likely as the general population to take long-term sick leave. These results, too, are conservative—they do not include analysis of overweight (as distinguished from obese) populations in these countries.[84]

Poor nutrition undermines a nation's health care system as well. Unlike the diseases of undernutrition, which often kill the young or inflict permanent and untreatable damage such as stunting or blindness, treatment of chronic illness often involves frequent use of the health care system. The overweight and obese in the Netherlands visit their physicians 20 percent and 40 percent more, respectively, than people of healthy weight. And obese people there were 2.5 times more likely to require drugs prescribed for cardiovascular and circulation disorders.[85]

The economic cost of these burdens to health care appears to be enormous. Comparing the prevalence of hypertension, heart disease, cancer, diabetes, gallstones, obesity, and food-borne illness among vegetarians and meat eaters in the United States, the Physicians Committee for

Responsible Medicine estimated total annual medical costs in 1995 related to meat consumption of between $29 billion and $61 billion. The costs would likely have been higher if stroke and other arterial diseases had been studied as well.[86]

Meanwhile, Dr. Colditz at Harvard has calculated the direct costs (hospital stays, medicine, treatment, and visits to the doctor) and indirect costs (reduced productivity, missed workdays, disability pensions) of obesity in the United States to be $118 billion annually, or nearly 12 percent of the nation's health care expenditures. (This is more than double the $47 billion in costs attributable to cigarette smoking in the United States.) Add to this sum the $33 billion spent on diet drugs and weight loss programs, together with the unmeasurable psychological costs from the social exclusion associated with being overweight, and the full cost of overeating begins to emerge.[87]

Whichever figure is used, such sums place an enormous drag on a nation's development. Money spent to counteract obesity or to reverse the damage done by meat consumption—health effects that are largely avoidable—cannot be used to address other social problems. In this sense, poor nutrition—like pollution, crime, or excessive military spending—has the potential to hobble or even unravel a nation's development gains.

The high cost of malnutrition poses particularly acute challenges for developing countries, which must tackle large caseloads of both infectious and chronic diseases on shoestring budgets. Many developing countries spend less than $25 per person annually on health care, compared with $4,000 in industrial nations. India and China, for example, spend $17 and $31, respectively, on health care.[88]

Treating chronic diseases in developing countries in the future will cost a great deal: WCRF/AICR researchers warn that without effective policies for cancer prevention, the cost of treating cancer in developing countries will rise 25-fold between 1985 and 2015. The cost of treating cancer alone may exceed the entire national budget for health care in many developing countries by then. Because chronic disease usually afflicts the wealthy—at least initially—in developing countries, and because the wealthy often wield disproportionate political clout, the pressure to give priority to treatment of chronic diseases will probably be strong. Those suffering from infectious disease—typically the poor—are likely to be left out.[89]

The broad costs of malnutrition extend still further, since malnutrition tends to reinforce the social inequalities that give rise to poor eating in the first place. Where hunger leads to high rates of infant mortality, for instance, population growth is often high, as couples have large families to offset likely losses of children. Such overcompensation further burdens poor families. At the other end of the nutritional spectrum, obesity can also keep people in poverty. Obese women in the United States generally have less education and less income than other women, and obese young adults are less likely to reach the same social class level as their peers. What's more, these disadvantages are handed down from generation to generation, as children learn poor eating habits from their parents.[90]

Nutrition First

Half of the world is malnourished, more than half of the world's burden of disease is likely linked to poor diet, and some of these diseases are spreading at an epidemic clip. The world is in the midst of a nutrition crisis, and its toll on human development is staggering, yet largely unrecognized. Reversing the trend toward worsening diets requires that nutrition, long treated as an afterthought by many national leaders, become a clear policy priority. For this to happen, policymakers need to see hunger and overeating as the product of human decisions—part societal and part individual—that government policies can influence.

The most urgent task facing policymakers is to attend to those who are hungry or deficient in micronutrients.

Distribution of food aid, supplementary feeding programs, and fortification of foods can all be launched quickly, often with great success. UNICEF and WHO, for example, set out early in the 1990s to eliminate iodine deficiency disorder, largely by persuading 47 nations to establish programs to iodize salt, thereby doubling the number of countries with this capacity. As a result, the global population at risk of IDD dropped from 29 percent to 13 percent between 1994 and 1997.[91]

A similar commitment could be made concerning iron, vitamin A, and other micronutrients, many of which can easily be added to foods. Such fortification is generally quite affordable at around 10¢ per beneficiary per year. (See Table 6.) Feeding programs require more fiscal effort, costing some $70–$100 per beneficiary annually. But especially for key populations like pregnant women and young children, the alternative—in terms of loss of life, loss of productivity, and increased health care costs—is likely to make such investments look like a bargain.[92]

Perhaps a greater bargain, and another initiative that can be quickly implemented, is the promotion of breast-feeding. Researchers calculated in the 1980s that effective breast-feeding campaigns could reduce illness from diarrhea by 8–20 percent and death from diarrhea by 24–27 percent during a baby's first six months. Some governments have gone a step further in encouraging breast-feeding: for example, Papua New Guinea only allows the sale of feeding bottles with a prescription. And the Baby-Friendly Hospital Initiative, a joint UNICEF and WHO program, facilitates breast-feeding by prohibiting the promotion of breast-milk substitutes in hospitals and permitting mothers and infants to room together.[93]

Interventions such as these, however, are not sufficient to end hunger. Eradicating hunger requires elimination of its root cause, which is often poverty. Job creation, affordable food pricing, microcredit, women's education, land redistribution—any number of diverse measures that reduce poverty and improve social services are likely to improve

TABLE 6

Costs of a Range of Nutrition Interventions

Intervention	Cost per Beneficiary per Year (dollars)
Micronutrient fortification	0.05-0.15
Micronutrient supplementation	0.20-1.70
Mass media education	0.20-2.00
Other education programs, such as breast-feeding promotion	5
Community-based programs such as home gardening and growth monitoring	5-10
Feeding programs (per 1,000 calories a day)	70-100

Source: See endnote 92.

nutrition. A 1999 study of malnutrition in 63 countries by the International Food Policy Research Institute found that social factors—health environment, women's education, and women's status—accounted for nearly three quarters of the reduction in malnutrition in these countries, with food availability per person an important fourth factor. Indeed, where governments are committed to improving social safety nets and ensuring gender equity, hunger has been substantially reduced or even contained.[94]

The Indian state of Kerala, for instance, subsidizes food shops, health care, and education, guaranteeing access to all, including women and rural inhabitants, two groups that often have the lowest incomes. This social safety net is credited with keeping the share of hungry children at 32 percent compared with 53 percent for India overall. Kerala's success is especially noteworthy given that economic growth and per capita incomes there are below the Indian average.[95]

Cuba is another example where commitment to meeting basic human needs has made hunger rare—even in the face of severe economic challenges. The collapse of the Soviet Union, Cuba's major trading partner, combined with an ongoing U.S. trade embargo, brought about food and fuel shortages, and the reduced caloric availability came just as reduced access to motorized transports increased expenditure of human energy. As a result, infant mortality and rates of low birthweight—among the lowest in North and South America—began to rise in some parts of the country. The government responded immediately by targeting children, the elderly, and pregnant women with nutritional assistance through school lunch programs and special ration privileges. This policy priority ensured that children, the elderly, and pregnant women were largely spared the worst effects of malnutrition during the years of food scarcity. Today, underweight among children, as well as infant mortality, has returned to among the lowest in the Americas. The government essentially recognized freedom from hunger as a basic human right, a concept that is enshrined in the U.N.'s Declaration of Human Rights but largely ignored by most governments.[96]

Similarly, strong commitment to public education and other social infrastructure in South Korea and Taiwan has opened wide access to economic opportunities, while land redistribution and heavy investment in agriculture—the leading economic sector in many developing countries—assured that rural prosperity was widespread and not limited to a few wealthy landowners. The result has been rapid and "shared" economic growth that has dampened income inequalities and kept poverty at bay. Especially in rural areas, where most of the world's hungry now live, improving agricultural credit, marketing, and distribution and targeting agricultural investment to small and middle-sized farms are often the fastest routes to eliminating poverty.[97]

Improving the well-being and nutritional status of the rural poor has been particularly difficult because development patterns since the Industrial Revolution have tended to favor cities—the centers of economic growth and political lobbies. This "urban bias," which prevails even in predominantly rural nations today, means that government budgets often favor projects that serve the urban elite, such as a few hi-tech hospitals, while neglecting rural health clinics or other basic services in the countryside.[98]

The growing ranks of the urban hungry require a different array of policy tools, including subsidized food shops, food-for-work (employment) programs, and childcare assistance for working mothers. Here it is important to keep the policy focus on the need to improve access to food, since urbanites generally grow a smaller share of their food than their rural cousins do. An especially effective tool for promoting access to food in cities is support of urban agriculture. Urban food gardens in Cuba, for example, which meet 30 percent of the vegetable demand in some cities, have prospered

Urban food gardens in Cuba meet 30 percent of the vegetable demand in some cities.

under government nurturing. Rights to vacant urban lots, provision of water, and promotion of farmers' markets have all helped to increase the supply of affordable vegetables in Cuban cities.[99]

Another effective strategy for reducing poverty and alleviating hunger is microcredit, the provision of tiny loans to the very poor, who typically cannot secure financing through conventional banks. These loans allow a basket weaver, for example, to boost income by buying supplies in bulk, or a farmer to produce additional food by investing in an irrigation system. Microcredit has been shown to boost income, and evidence suggests that microcredit programs can be administered in a way that directly targets nutritional improvement. In particular, directing loans to women is likely to raise nutritional levels. A 1998 study of Bangladeshi participants in the Grameen Bank, the world's largest microcredit bank, found that participation had a significant positive effect on child nutrition "as long as women rather than men received the loans," simply because women are more disposed to direct increased income to household needs.[100]

In addition, loans are most likely to raise nutritional levels when accompanied by education about health and nutrition. A "Credit with Education" program initiated in Ghana by the international group Freedom from Hunger coupled lending with education about breast-feeding, child feeding, diarrhea prevention, immunization, and family planning. A three-year follow-up study documented improved health and nutrition practices, fewer and shorter-lived episodes of food shortages, and dramatic improvements in childrens' nutrition among the participants compared with the control group.[101]

The Ghanaian program is an example of an increasingly popular approach to nutritional intervention known as community-based nutrition. In contrast to traditional top-down approaches, community programs are decentralized grassroots-based efforts that involve the affected population in every facet of planning and execution. And where possible, they are careful to involve local leaders or authority figures. Indeed, a 1996 U.N. assessment of nutrition interventions underlines the importance of community involvement: "... it is the organization of activities and the process of carrying them out—how and by whom—not so much their content as such, that is of crucial importance."[102]

In the Gambia, Save the Children Federation USA and the Gambian Ministry of Health and Social Welfare targeted the highly respected women elders of the matriarchal Kabilo tribe with information on child-feeding practices, basic hygiene, and maternal health care, and maternal and child mortality dropped dramatically. A more extensive, country-wide program in the Philippines, called BIDANI, asks mothers and village leaders to identify the sources of malnutrition in their villages, and involves them in orientation, training, and planning for nutritional interventions—interventions that local residents decide are best for their communities. The latest program assessment indicates that after 12 months, 82 percent of enrolled children moved to a higher nutritional status. The sense of ownership that is central to a community-based approach to nutrition gives participants greater incentive to work for success, and to ensure that the program is sustained over the long term.[103]

Just as community nutrition programs build upon existing village structures, smart nutrition policy will incorporate nutrition objectives into existing government social programs. Health, education, and agricultural extension programs already reach deep into nutritionally vulnerable populations through existing networks of clinics, schools, and rural development offices. Yet governments are missing many opportunities to exploit these synergies. Expansion of their responsibilities to include nutrition intervention would be a natural and cost-effective way to promote good nutrition. Clinic staff could promote breast-feeding, for example, and extension agents could encourage home gardening, thereby maximizing the return on NGO and government social investments.[104]

The international community shares responsibility for eliminating hunger by assisting national governments or by ensuring that international institutions promote and respect food security. International aid to agriculture dropped nearly 50 percent in real terms between 1986 and 1996, while total development aid from the world's wealthiest nations dropped to just 0.22 percent of their collective gross national product—the lowest level ever and far lower than the United Nations target of 0.7 percent. Debt relief, development aid, and assistance for family planning programs—the latter representing one of the most cost-effective means to improve incomes, health, and the lives of women and their children—are among the international initiatives that can alleviate poverty and reduce hunger. There also remains a need to restructure free trade agreements so that they adequately protect the right of countries to support rural livelihoods and food production for domestic markets. This support must be differentiated from subsidies for export-oriented production, which are currently discouraged under international trade law.[105]

In nations where overeating is a problem, or rapidly

becoming one, policymakers require a different set of policy tools. Technofixes attract great attention: liposuction is now the leading form of cosmetic surgery in the United States, at 400,000 operations per year; designer foods such as olestra promise worry-free consumption of nutritionally empty snacks; and laboratories scurry to find the human "fat gene" in an effort to engineer a way out of obesity. But such quick fixes typically fail to confront the behavioral patterns, such as poor eating habits and sedentary lifestyles, that underlie obesity. Indeed, while experts agree that more research is needed to determine the recipe for sustainable weight loss, studies to date identify three elements common to people who lose weight and keep it off: they eat a low-fat diet, they watch their total calorie intake, and they regularly engage in vigorous, physical activity. These common sense ingredients stand in sharp contrast to today's diet fads. Renewed attention to diverse, balanced diets and active lifestyles will require education—with a focus on prevention—and modification of the food environment.[106]

A high-payoff venue for nutrition education is schools, where children—whose eating habits are still being formed—are gathered in one place, and meals are generally served. In Singapore, for example, the Trim and Fit Scheme has reduced obesity among children by 33 to 50 percent, depending on the age group, through changes in school catering and increased nutrition and physical education for teachers and children. Programs like this can have lasting effects. In the United States, the Child and Adolescent Trial for Cardiovascular Health targeted children from diverse socioeconomic and cultural backgrounds in grades three through five with additional nutrition and physical education, and it yielded behavioral changes that persisted at least into adolescence: a three-year follow-up, without further intervention, showed dietary fat intake to be substantially lower and daily vigorous activity substantially higher in participating children than in control groups.[107]

At a more basic level, schools can model healthy nutrition and lifestyles by meeting basic standards for food and exercise. American schools were only recently—in 1994— required to comply with the USDA's national dietary guidelines, and surveys show that most still provide meals that are excessive in fat and low in fiber. At the same time, only 25 percent of American high schools offered daily physical education classes in 1995, down from 42 percent in 1991. Reversing the alarming rise in childhood obesity in the United States will require attention to nutritional fundamentals such as caloric balance and dietary diversity.[108]

An especially effective approach to nutrition education is "hands-on" learning, which allows students to cook and taste healthy food, critique food advertisements, and read nutrition labels. One example of this philosophy is found in Berkeley, California, where schools have started vegetable gardens to help children learn about food and nutrition, and to supply some of the food for school cafeterias, which were required in 1999 to begin serving all-organic lunches. Similarly, the "Get Cooking!" project in the United Kingdom has taught healthy cooking and other home economics skills to school children since 1993, and has found that "children will bring the knowledge home and demand nutritious and tasty home-cooked meals from their parents."[109]

Only 25 percent of American high schools offered daily physical education classes in 1995.

Households, of course, are also a natural venue for nutrition education. Children learn some of their most important lessons about eating at home, and these lessons can be positive. Research shows that participants in family-based weight control programs—in which children and parents learn and practice healthy habits together—are more successful in losing weight over the long term than participants in programs that target individuals. Family-based nutrition education can also be a useful model for preventing unhealthy weight gain in the first place, before it becomes a deeply rooted problem that is costly and difficult to eradicate.[110]

Nutrition education is especially critical for doctors, nurses, and other health care providers, who are in a key position to educate patients about the links between diet and health. Doctors unfamiliar with the impact of diet on health respond only to the consequences of poor nutrition rather than to early warning signs that suggest the need for a change in diet, increase in physical activity, or other preventive measures. In the United States, only 23 percent of medical schools required that students take a separate course in nutrition in 1994—a benchmark that could be raised.[111]

For society at large, mass education campaigns may be needed to change long-standing nutritional habits. One of the most successful national nutrition education campaigns was carried out by Finland in the 1970s and 1980s to reduce the country's high incidence of coronary heart disease. Government-sponsored media campaigns, national dietary guidelines, and regulations on food labeling were among the diverse educational tools used to drive home the nutritional message. This broad, high-profile approach—it also advocated an end to smoking, and involved groups as diverse as farmers and the Finnish Heart Association—slashed mortality from coronary heart disease by 65 percent between 1969–71 and 1995. About half of the drop is credited to the lower levels of cholesterol induced by the nutrition education campaign.[112]

Less ambitious but still strategically focused approaches to nutrition education can also provide a large payoff. A consumers' organization in the United States reports that more than two thirds of all shoppers are "very interested" in increasing their consumption of fresh fruits and vegetables. But the same share of shoppers admitted that they did not know how to prepare or eat these foods—and therefore did not buy them. Supermarkets and others in the food business could help by teaching consumers the skills needed for healthy diets.[113]

A nutritionally literate public will begin to demand different foods, to which the food industry may respond with wider offerings of low-fat, whole-grain, and other healthier selections. Governments can help markets to promote good nutrition by regulating nutritional information that is displayed on food products. Such a system will have greater credibility, however, if it not only provides positive nutrition information, but also requires equally prominent warning labels on unhealthy foods. In Finland, the government now requires "heavily salted" to appear on foods high in sodium, while allowing low-sodium foods to bear the label "reduced salt content."[114]

Similarly, governments may need to regulate harmful nutritional information, especially the advertising of nutritionally poor foods. Sweden and Norway, for instance, do not allow any advertising aimed at children under 12, while the Flemish region of Belgium prohibits advertising five minutes before or after children's programs. And more than a dozen European countries have voluntary, self-regulating codes of conduct for advertising aimed at children.[115]

Is Ronald McDonald really so different from Joe Camel?

Some nutrition advocates, including Yale professor Kelly Brownell, have argued that regulating advertising of junk foods is similar to curbing the promotion of cigarettes: both industries target children in an effort to win lifelong customers, both make products that kill in great numbers, and both drive up health care costs substantially. Does it make sense to allow nutrition-poor foods to be promoted and sold freely while tobacco is increasingly regulated? Is Ronald McDonald really so different from Joe Camel?[116]

As support for healthy eating grows, consumption of nutrient-poor foods can be further reduced using fiscal tools. Brownell advocates adoption of a tax on food based on the nutrient value per calorie. Fatty and sugary foods low in nutrients and loaded with calories would be taxed the most, while fruits and vegetables might escape taxation entirely. The idea is to discourage consumption of unhealthy foods— and to raise revenue to promote healthier alternatives, nutrition education, or exercise programs. While controversial, adoption of such a tax perhaps becomes more politically palatable as the price of many nutritionally poor foods falls in real terms. Between 1978 and 1999 in the United States, for example, the real price of soda fell by 26 percent and the real price of ground beef declined by 31 percent, while fresh vegetables and fruits increased in price by 27 percent and 67 percent, respectively. This initiative would best be accompanied by efforts in mass public education to protect low-income people, whose diets are especially high in nutritionally poor foods, from adverse effects.[117]

Brownell's tax proposal is especially attractive in light of clear evidence that price has a powerful impact on dietary choice. A 1994 study of cafeteria food purchases demonstrates this. For the study, the number of fruit choices was doubled, selections of salad fixings were tripled, and the price of fruit and salads was cut by half. The results: purchases of fruit and salad tripled over the test period, even as total food purchases remained the same. Subsequent cafeteria and vending machine studies have produced similar results, and accord with consumer research showing price to be among the highest criteria used to make food-purchasing decisions.[118]

A final part of reshaping the food environment is recultivating an appreciation of food as a cultural and nutritional treasure. As the consumer culture invades the realm of eating, brand allegiance has triumphed over concerns of nutrition and health and mega-meals have replaced the ethic of sufficiency. Groups like the Slow Food Movement, based in Italy, and the Oldways Preservation and Exchange Trust in the United States offer a postmodern critique of today's culinary norm by promoting a return to the art of cooking traditional foods and of socializing around food. Their work, which targets chefs as well as consumers, is the kind of cultural intervention that could help more people shift to a healthy diet, similar to the change in consciousness that encouraged a shift away from smoking in the United States. Government encouragement of these groups, perhaps through assistance with marketing and promotional activities, would insure that this important work benefits everyone, not just elites.[119]

Whatever the nutritional policies chosen, they ultimately work best when partnered with complementary initiatives in other sectors of national development. The idea is not new—the League of Nations recommended to member states in the 1940s a "marriage between agriculture and health" that would unite officials from food, economic, and health ministries to make nutrition policy. Norway is one of the few countries to follow this advice: its interministerial National Nutrition Council dates back to the 1940s and considers agricultural self-sufficiency, rural development, environmental conservation, and world food security—in addition to health and diet—when making nutrition policy.[120]

Today, an even greater range of expertise may be needed to craft nutrition policy. The ministry of public works, for example, could be a key player in a campaign to reduce micronutrient deficiencies: a cleaner water supply would reduce the incidence of intestinal parasites, which hamper the body's capacity to absorb micronutrients. Likewise, a broader cast of advocates is needed to fight the poor diet and sedentary lifestyle that produce obesity. Transportation officials might be enlisted to promote bicycle commuting, ministers of education and culture could discourage TV watching, and the agriculture ministry might promote appreciation of food as a nutritional and cultural treasure.

In an age of unprecedented global prosperity, it is paradoxical—and wholly unnecessary—that malnutrition should exist on such a massive scale. Indeed, poorly nourished people are a sign of "progress" gone awry: prosperity has either bypassed them and left them hungry, or saturated them to the point of overindulgence. But a nation's development path is the product of human choices, and can therefore be redirected. By providing access to nutritionally sound food for all, governments can shape a social evolution that can truly be called development.

Notes

1. Clark Spencer Larsen, "Biological Changes in Human Populations with Agriculture," *Annual Review of Anthropology*, 1995; idem, University of North Carolina at Chapel Hill, discussion with Brian Halweil, 14 December 1999.

2 . Larsen, "Biological Changes," op. cit. note 1.

3. Ibid.

4. Ibid.

5. Half the world from World Health Organization (WHO), *World Health Report 1998* (Geneva: 1998); 1.2 billion overweight and underweight are Worldwatch estimates, from United Nations (U.N.), Administrative Committee on Coordination, Sub-Committee on Nutrition (UN ACC/SCN), "Fourth Report on the World Nutrition Situation" (draft) (New York: July 1999), from WHO, *Obesity: Preventing and Managing the Global Epidemic, Report of a WHO Consultation on Obesity* (Geneva: 1997), from K.M. Flegal et al., "Overweight and Obesity in the United States, Prevalence and Trends, 1960–1994," *International Journal of Obesity*, August 1998, and from Rafael Flores, Research Fellow, International Food Policy Research Institute (IFPRI), Washington, DC, e-mail to Brian Halweil, 5 November 1999 and discussion with Gary Gardner, 3 February 2000; micronutrient deficiency from UN ACC/SCN, op. cit. this note; Table 1 from UN ACC/SCN, op. cit. this note, from WHO, *Obesity*, op. cit. this note, from Flegal et al., op. cit. this note, and from Flores, op. cit. this note; half of modern-day Georgians from Flegal et al., op. cit. this note.

6. Half or more of the world's burden of disease based on John Mason, Department of International Health and Development, Tulane University, New Orleans, letter to Brian Halweil, 16 September 1999, Christopher J.L. Murray and Alan D. Lopez, eds., *The Global Burden of Disease* (Cambridge, MA: Harvard University Press, 1996), and Alan D. Lopez, Harvard University, discussion with Brian Halweil, 15 August 1999; more than 5 million children from WHO, "Malnutrition Worldwide," <www.who.int/nut>, viewed 20 December 1999.

7. Obesity costs from Graham Colditz, Harvard School of Public Health, "The Economic Costs of Obesity and Inactivity," unpublished manuscript; India from Anthony R. Measham and Meera Chatterjee, "Wasting Away: The Crisis of Malnutrition in India" (Washington, DC: World Bank, 1999); women from UN ACC/SCN, op. cit. note 5,· and from U.N. Food and Agriculture Organization (FAO), "Women Feed the World," prepared for World Food Day, 16 October 1998 (Rome: 1998).

8. Diabetes from International Diabetes Federation (IDF), "Diabetes Around the World" (Brussels: 1998), and <www.idf.org>, viewed 14 July 1999.

9.   Kerala from C. R. Soman, Professor of Nutrition, College of Medicine, University of Kerala, e-mail to Brian Halweil, 29 October 1999; Cuba from Dr. Jorge Dotres, Minister of Health, Republic of Cuba, presentation at Johns Hopkins School of Public Health, Baltimore, MD, 1998.

10. Advertising in United States from Anthony E. Gallo, "Food Advertising in the United States," in Elizabeth Frazao, ed., *America's Eating Habits: Changes and Consequences* (Washington, DC: United States Department of Agriculture (USDA), Economic Research Service (ERS), April 1999), and advertising in Austria, Belgium, and France from NTC Publications, *European Marketing Pocket Book*, 1999 Edition (Oxfordshire, U.K.: 1998); more than half of advertising from Consumers International, *A Spoonful of Sugar, Television Food Advertising Aimed at Children: An International Comparative Survey* (London: 1996); overweight and obesity among Americans from Flegal et al., op. cit. note 5.

11. Susan Horton, "The Economics of Nutrition Interventions" (draft, April 1999) in R.D. Semba, ed., *Nutrition and Health in Developing Countries* (Totowa, NJ: Humana Press, forthcoming).

12. Table 2 from FAO, *The State of Food Insecurity in the World* (Rome: 1999); WHO, *Obesity*, op. cit. note 5; Flegal et al., op. cit. note 5.

13. Corinne Cataldo et al., *Nutrition and Diet Therapy: Principles and Practices* (Belmont, CA: Wadsworth Publishing, 1999).

14. Ibid.; traditional diets from a multiyear international conference series, "Public Health Implications of Traditional Diets," organized by Oldways Preservation & Exchange Trust, Cambridge, MA, <www.oldwayspt.com>, viewed 31 January 2000.

15. FAO, op cit. note 12; Lisa Smith, *Can FAO's Measure of Chronic Undernourishment Be Strengthened?* Food Consumption and Nutrition Division (FCND) Discussion Paper No. 44 (Washington, DC: IFPRI, May 1998).

16. Table 3 from UN ACC/SCN, op. cit. note 5.

17. UN ACC/SCN, "Fourth Report on the World Nutrition Situation," op. cit. note 5.

18. Lawrence Haddad, Marie T. Ruel, and James L. Garrett, "Are Urban Poverty and Undernutrition Growing? Some Newly Assembled Evidence," Food Consumption and Nutrition Division (FCND) Discussion Paper No. 63 (Washington, DC: IFPRI, April 1999).

19. USDA, "Household Food Security in the United States, 1995-1998" (Advance Report) (Washington, DC: July 1999); Graham Riches, ed., *First World Hunger* (New York: St. Martin's Press, 1997).

20. WHO, *Obesity*, op. cit. note 5; BMI is calculated as a person's weight in kilos divided by the square of height in meters. Thus, a person standing 1.78 meters (5 feet, 10 inches) tall and weighing 80 kilos (175 pounds) has a BMI of 25, and is considered overweight; at 95 kilos (210 pounds), the same person would be considered obese.

21. Flegal et al., op. cit. note 5; childhood overweight and obesity from Rajen Anand, introductory presentation to "Childhood Obesity: Causes and Prevention," symposium sponsored by USDA, Center for Nutrition Policy and Promotion, Washington, DC, 27 October 1998; obesity in Europe from WHO, *Obesity*, op. cit. note 5.

22. U.N. survey from Flores, op. cit. note 5; China data from Catherine Geissler, "China: The Soya Pork Dilemma," *Proceedings of the Nutrition Society*, May 1999, and from Barry M. Popkin et al., "Body Weight Patterns among the Chinese: Results from the 1989 and 1991 China Health and Nutrition Surveys," *American Journal of Public Health*, May 1995; Brazil and Colombia from WHO, *Obesity*, op. cit. note 5; overweight exceeding underweight from Flores, op. cit. note 5.

23. Three micronutrients from UN ACC/SCN, op. cit. note 5.

24. WHO, "World Health Organization Sets Out to Eliminate Iodine Deficiency Disorder," press release, 2 pages (Geneva: 25 May 1999); Vitamin A from UN ACC/SCN, op. cit. note 5.

25. UN ACC/SCN, op. cit. note 5; Flores, op. cit. note 5.

26. Exclusive breast-feeding in Latin America from ibid.; UNICEF recommendation from Ted Greiner, Section for International Maternal and Child Health, Uppsala University, Sweden, e-mail to authors, 21 October 1999; exclusive breast-feeding in North America from Alan Ryan, Ross Products Division, Abbott Laboratories, Inc., Cleveland, OH, fax to authors, 26 October 1999.

27. Industrial-nation calorie breakdown from World Cancer Research Fund and the American Institute for Cancer Research (WCRF/AICR), *Food, Nutrition, and the Prevention of Cancer: A Global Perspective* (Washington, DC: AICR, 1997); refined grains from Judy Putnam and Shirley Gerrior, "Trends in the U.S. Food Supply, 1970-97," in Frazao, ed., op. cit. note 10; french fries and potato chips from Linda Scott Kantor, "A Comparison of the U.S. Food Supply with the Food Guide Pyramid Recommendations," in Frazao, op. cit. this note.

28. Americans from Dirk Johnson, "Snacking Today: Any Time and Anywhere," *New York Times*, 30 July 1999; U.K. from John Willman, "Appetite for Snack Food Soars to $3.6 Billion a Year," *Financial Times*, 22 September 1999.

29. Home-made meals from Dave Jenkins, NPD Group, Inc., e-mail to Brian Halweil, 23 August 1999; McKinsey & Co. consumer behavior study cited in Dave Gussow, "Will Tomorrow's Consumers Really Buy House Brimming With Smart Appliances?" *Environmental News Network*, 23 June 1999.

30. Amartya Sen, *Poverty and Famines: An Essay on Entitlement and Deprivation* (New York: Oxford University Press, 1981); 80 percent of all malnourished children from Lisa Smith, *Can FAO's Measure of Chronic Undernourishment Be Strengthened?* FCND Discussion Paper No. 44 (Washington, DC: IFPRI, May 1998); Lisa C. Smith and Lawrence Haddad, "Explaining Child Malnutrition in Developing Countries: A Cross-Country Analysis," FCND Discussion Paper No. 60 (Washington, DC: IFPRI, April 1999); UNICEF, *State of the World's Children* (New York: 1998).

31. FAO, op. cit. note 7.

32. Ibid.

33. Ross M. Welch, Gerald F. Combs, Jr., and John M. Duxbury, "Toward a 'Greener' Revolution," *Issues in Science and Technology*, fall 1997; grain and pulse consumption in South Asia from FAO, *FAOSTAT*, electronic database, <apps.fao.org>, updated 9 December 1999.

34. Gordon R. Conway and Edward B. Barbier, *After the Green Revolution: Sustainable Agriculture for Development* (London: Earthscan Publications, 1990) Mexico from Susan George, "Latin America: Going to Extremes," in Douglas H. Boucher, *The Paradox of Plenty: Hunger in a Bountiful World* (Oakland, CA: Food First Books, 1999).

35. Relationship between land distribution, rural poverty, and hunger from Klaus Deininger and Lin Squire, "New Ways of Looking at Old Issues: Inequality and Growth," *Journal of Development Economics*, December 1998, and from Daniel Maxwell and Keith Wiebe, "Land Tenure and Food Security: A Review of Concepts, Evidence, and Methods," LTC Research Paper 129 (Madison: Land Tenure Center, University of Wisconsin, January 1998); India from Timothy Besley and Robin Burgess, "Land Reform, Poverty Reduction and Growth: Evidence from India," Research Report, Department of Economics, London School of Economics, 8 July 1998.

36. Giovanni Andrea Cornia, Richard Jolly, and Frances Stewart eds., *Adjustment with a Human Face* (Oxford: Clarendon Press, 1988); Lance Taylor and Ute Pieper, *Reconciling Economic Reform and Sustainable Human Development: Social Consequences of Neo-Liberalism*, U.N. Development Programme (UNDP), Office of Development Studies, Discussion Paper Series (UNDP: New York, 1996); Nancy Alexander, "Remaking the World Bank and the International Monetary Fund," in *Hunger in a Global Economy* (Silver Spring, MD: Bread for the World Institute, 1997); *The All-Too-Visible Hand: A Five-Country Look at the Long and Destructive Reach of the IMF* (Washington, DC: Development Gap, April 1999).

37. Chile, Paraguay, and Guatemala from Maxwell and Wiebe, op. cit. note 35; benefits of food exports from Peter Uvin, *The International Organization of Hunger* (London: Kegan Paul International, 1994), from Lori Ann Thrupp, *Bittersweet Harvest for Global Supermarkets: Challenges in Latin America's Agricultural Export Boom* (Washington, DC: World Resources Institute (WRI), August 1995), from Walden Bello, "The WTO's Big Losers," *Far Eastern Economic Review*, 24 June 1999, and from Frances Moore Lappé et al., *World Hunger: Twelve Myths* (San Francisco: Grove Press, 1998).

38. Kevin Watkins, "Agricultural Trade and Food Security" (London: Oxfam, May 1996); Per Pinstrup-Andersen and Marc J. Cohen, "An Overview of the Future Global Food Situation," prepared for the Millennial Symposium on "Feeding a Planet," sponsored by and held at the Cosmos Club, Washington, DC, 12 February 1999; Sophia Murphy, "Trade and Food Security: An Assessment of the Uruguay Round Agreement on Agriculture" (London: Catholic Institute for International Relations, 1999); transitory effects from Marc Cohen, IFPRI, discussion with Brian Halweil, 12 December 1999.

39. Karen Lehman, "The Great Train Robbery of 1996" (Minneapolis, MN: Institute for Agriculture and Trade Policy, 25 June 1996); Watkins, op. cit. note 38.

40. Marc J. Cohen and Torsten Feldbruegge, *Acute Nutrition Crises and Violent Conflict* (Washington, DC: IFPRI, forthcoming).

41. Table 4 adapted from Barry M. Popkin, Department of Nutrition, University of North Carolina at Chapel Hill, "Urbanization, Lifestyle Changes, and the Nutrition Transition," unpublished manuscript, 11 August 1998.

42. Marion Nestle et al., "Behavioral and Social Influences on Food Choice," *Nutrition Reviews*, May 1998; B.J. Rolls and E.A. Bell, "Intake of Fat and Carbohydrate: Role of Energy Density," *European Journal of Clinical Nutrition*, April 1999; J.E. Blundell and J.I. MacDiarmid, "Fat as a Risk Factor for Overconsumption: Satiation, Satiety, and Patterns of Eating," *Journal of American Dietetic Association*, July 1997.

43. Barry M. Popkin, "The Nutrition Transition and Its Health Implications in Lower-Income Countries," *Public Health Nutrition*, January 1998.

44. Adam Drewnowski and Barry M. Popkin, "The Nutrition Transition: New Trends in the Global Diet," *Nutrition Reviews*, February 1997; Geissler, op. cit. note 22.

45. Share of Chinese households from X. Guo, T.A. Mroz, B.M. Popkin, and F. Zhai, "Structural Changes in the Impact of Income on Food Consumption in China, 1989–93," *Economic Development and Cultural Change* (in press); simultaneous under- and overweight from C.M. Doak, L. Adair, C.

Monteiro, and B.M. Popkin, "Overweight and Underweight Co-exists in Brazil, China, and Russia," University of North Carolina at Chapel Hill, unpublished manuscript, 1999. The authors note that the explanation for this co-existence within households is probably related to gender bias in food distribution and/or different levels of energy expenditure, though additional research is required.

46. Income level required for a given diet, and Japan and China comparison, from Drewnowski and Popkin, op. cit. note 44; Figure 1 from USDA, *Production, Supply, and Distribution*, electronic database, Washington, DC, updated December 1999.

47. Urban share of global population from Molly O'Meara, "Exploring a New Vision for Cities," in Lester Brown et al., *State of the World 1999* (New York: W.W. Norton & Company, 1999).

48. Drewnowski and Popkin, op. cit. note 44; Marie T. Ruel et al., "Urban Challenges to Food and Nutrition Security: A Review of Food Security, Health, and Caregiving in the Cities," FCND Discussion Paper No. 51, IFPRI, (Washington, DC: October 1998).

49. Barry M. Popkin, University of North Carolina at Chapel Hill, discussion with authors, 5 September 1999; Henry Chu, "Now Meat Is Raising Red Flags in China," *Los Angeles Times*, 27 July 1998.

50. Ruel et al., op. cit. note 48; rise of processed foods in industrial nations from J. Mauron, "Effects of Processed Foods on Food Consumption Patterns in Industrialized Countries," *Bibliographia Nutrition and Dieta*, February 1989.

51. Popkin, op. cit. note 43; share of population engaged in agriculture from FAO, op. cit. note 33.

52. Chinese overweight levels from Geissler, op. cit. note 22; Popkin, op. cit. note 43.

53. Countertrend from Carlos A. Monteiro et al., "Shifting Obesity Trends in Brazil," *European Journal of Clinical Nutrition* (in press), from Popkin, op. cit. note 43, and from Soowon Kim, Soojae Moon, and Barry M. Popkin, "The Nutrition Transition in South Korea," *American Journal of Clinical Nutrition* (in press); ethnic obesity from Flegal et al., op. cit. note 5.

54. Nestle et al., op. cit. note 42; Gallo, op. cit. note 10; Austria, Belgium, and France from NTC Publications, op. cit. note 10; Goeff Tansey and Tony Worsley, *The Food System: A Guide* (London: Earthscan Publications, 1995).

55. Ad spending and sales from Nestle et al., op. cit. note 42; infant formula from Naomi Baumslag and Dia L. Michels, *Milk, Money, and Madness: The Culture and Politics of Breastfeeding* (Westport, CT.: Bergin and Garvey,

1995) and Ministry of Foreign Affairs, *Nutrition: Interaction of Food, Health, and Care, Sectoral and Theme Policy Document of Development Cooperation*, No. 10 (The Hague: Government of the Netherlands, September 1998).

56. Consumers International, op. cit. note 10; U.S. fast-food ads from Gallo, op. cit. note 10; McDonald's and Coca-Cola from *Advertising Age*, <www.adage.com/dataplace>, viewed 5 October 1999.

57. Targeting of children and general studies from Nestle et al., op. cit. note 42; study on fourth- and fifth-graders from Victor C. Strasburger, *Adolescents and the Media* (Thousand Oaks, CA: Sage Publications 1995); life-long craving from Nestle et al., op. cit. note 42, and from L.L. Birch, "Development of Food Acceptance Patterns in the First Years of Life," *Proceedings of Nutrition Society*, November 1998.

58. Tansey and Worsley, op. cit. note 54; John Connor, Purdue University, discussion with Brian Halweil, 23 August 1999.

59. Michael Jacobson, Center for Science in the Public Interest (CSPI), discussion with Brian Halweil, 8 September 1999; Putnam and Gerrior, op. cit. note 27.

60. Manufacturer's promotions from Tansey and Worsley, op. cit. note 54; Pepsi from Constance L. Hayes, "An Aisle Unto Itself?" *New York Times*, 31 July 1999; 10 percent from Constance L. Hayes, discussion with Brian Halweil, 30 September 1999.

61. Anna White, "The Cola-ized Classroom," *Multinational Monitor*, January/February 1999; franchises in American schools from Claire Hope Cummings, "Entertainment Food," *The Ecologist*, January/February 1999.

62. Michael F. Jacobson, "Liquid Candy: How Soft Drinks are Harming Americans' Health" (Washington, DC: CSPI, October 1998); Brian Wansink, "Can Package Size Accelerate Usage Volume?" *Journal of Marketing*, July 1996; Lisa R. Young and Marion Nestle, "Variation in Perceptions of a 'Medium' Food Portion: Implications for Dietary Guidance," *Journal of the American Dietetic Association*, April 1998.

63. Marion Nestle, "Food Lobbies, the Food Pyramid, and US Nutrition Policy," *International Journal of Health Services*, March 1993; Dairy Council from Sue Markgraf, Dairy Management Inc., discussion with Brian Halweil, 23 September 1999, and from Vicki Urcuyo, Food and Nutrition Service, USDA, discussion with Brian Halweil, 12 December 1999.

64. Tim Lang, Professor of Food Policy, Thames Valley University, London, Michael Heasman and Jillian Pitt, "Food, Globalisation and a New Public Health Agenda," unpublished manuscript, July 1999.

65. Fast-food ads and nutrition education from Gallo, op. cit. note 10;

Kellogg's from Michael F. Jacobson, CSPI, Washington, DC, discussion with Brian Halweil, 26 October 1999; Kelly Brownell quote from Bonnie Liebman, "The Pressure to Eat," *Nutrition Action Healthletter* (CSPI), July/August 1998; Coca-Cola Company, *1997 Annual Report* (Atlanta: 1998).

66. Coca-Cola Company, *1998 Annual Report* (Atlanta: 1999); four of five McDonald's from Brian Breuhaus, "Risky Business?" *Restaurant Business*, 1 November 1998; Steven A. Neff et al., *Globalization of the Processed Foods Market* (Washington, DC: USDA, ERS, October 1996).

67. Table 5 based on the following: cancer from WCRF/AICR, op. cit. note 27; coronary heart disease from A.M. Wolf and G.A. Colditz, "Current Estimates of the Economic Costs of Obesity in the United States," *Obesity Research*, March 1998; adult-onset (Type II) diabetes from WHO, *Obesity*, op. cit. note 5; childhood blindness from Dr. Alfred Sommer, School of Public Health, Johns Hopkins University, Baltimore, MD, discussion with Brian Halweil, 2 November 1999; mental retardation from Ministry of Foreign Affairs, op. cit. note. 55, and from WHO, *World Health Report*, op. cit. note 5.

68. Mason, op. cit. note 6; John Mason notes that the 22 percent for hunger and 18 percent for micronutrient deficiencies cannot simply be added, due to overlap in the population affected, as well as possible synergies between the two conditions; original study is Murray and Lopez, eds., op. cit. note 6. The original study uses the term Disability-Adjusted Life Year (DALY), and defines one DALY as "one lost year of healthy life"; Dr. Lopez's estimate from his discussion with Brian Halweil, op. cit. note 6.

69. UN ACC/SCN, op. cit. note 5.

70. D.J.P. Barker, *Mothers, Babies, and Disease in Later Life* (London: British Medical Journal Publishing, 1994).

71. UN ACC/SCN, op. cit. note 5; Barker quoted in Alan Berg, "Furthermore...," *New and Noteworthy in Nutrition* (World Bank), 12 June 1999; 54 percent from Sonya Rabeneck, UN ACC/SCN, e-mail to authors, 5 October 1999.

72. Ministry of Foreign Affairs, op. cit. note 55.

73. UN ACC/SCN, op. cit. note 5; mental impairment *in utero* from Rafael Flores, IFPRI, Washington, DC, e-mail to authors, 14 October 1999.

74. "Recommendations to Prevent and Control Iron Deficiency in the United States," *Morbidity and Mortality Weekly Report*, 3 April 1998; Mary Murray, "Ads Raise Questions About Milk and Bones," *New York Times*, 14 September 1999; T. Remer and F. Manz, "Estimation of the Renal Net Acid Excretion by Adults Consuming Diets Containing Variable Amounts of Protein," *American Journal of Clinical Nutrition*, June 1994; D. Feskanich et al., "Milk, Dietary Calcium, and Bone Fractures in Women: A 12-Year Prospective Study," *American Journal of Public Health*, June 1997.

75. Popkin, op. cit. note 43.

76. China Health Survey from J. Chen et al., *Diet, Lifestyle, and Mortality in China: a Study of the Characteristics of 65 Chinese Counties* (Oxford: Oxford University Press, 1990), and from T. Colin Campbell, "Associations of Diet and Disease: A Comprehensive Study of Health Characteristics in China," presented at conference on "Social Consequences of Chinese Economic Reforms," Harvard University, Fairbank Center on East Asian Studies, Cambridge, MA, 23–24 May 1997; Framingham Study from Susan Brink, "Unlocking the Heart's Secrets," *U.S. News & World Report*, 7 September 1998.

77. WHO, *Obesity*, op. cit. note 5; industrial-nation mortality from WHO, op. cit. note 5, and from U.S. Centers for Disease Control and Prevention, National Center for Health Statistics, <www.cdc.gov/nchs/fastats/ deaths.htm>, viewed 31 January 2000; Wolf and Colditz, op. cit. note 67; WCRF/ AICR, op. cit. note 27.

78. WHO, *Obesity*, op. cit. note 5; D.C. Neiman et al., "Influence of Obesity on Immune Function," *Journal of American Dietetic Association*, March 1999.

79. IDF, op. cit. note 8; Ginger Thompson, "With Obesity in Children Rising, More Get Adult Type of Diabetes," *New York Times*, 14 December 1998; Elizabeth Frazao, "The High Costs of Poor Eating Habits in the United States," in Frazao, op. cit. note 10.

80. IDF, op. cit. note 8; WCRF/AICR, op. cit. note 27; Popkin, op. cit. note 43.

81. World Bank study from Ministry of Foreign Affairs, op. cit. note 55; Spain and Indonesia from Beryl Levinger, *Nutrition, Health, and Education for All* (New York: UNDP, 1994); Philippines study from M.E. Mendez and L.S. Adair, "Severity and Timing of Stunting in Infancy and Performance on IQ and School Achievement Tests in Late Childhood," *Journal of Nutrition*, August 1999. Equally interesting, this Filipino study found that the effects of stunting were reduced if an improved diet in later childhood allowed the infants' growth to catch up with their peers; however, the previously stunted children still performed more poorly than their peers who were never stunted.

82. Horton, op. cit. note 11.

83. Productivity losses ibid.; analysis of Horton's work from Jay Ross and Susan Horton, *Economic Consequences of Iron Deficiency* (Ottawa, Ontario: Micronutrient Initiative, 1998). Horton's estimates are conservative for several other reasons as well. They are based only on market economic activi-

ty, so they do not include socially valuable nonmarket losses. They also assume the maximum possible overlap among deficiencies—a country with 10 million hungry and 3 million iron-deficient persons is assumed to have 10 million malnourished—so estimates of productivity loss are minimums. India from Measham and Chatterjeem, op. cit. note 7.

84. U.S. statistics from Wolf and Colditz, op. cit. note 67, and from Anne Wolf, University of Virginia, Charlottesville, VA, discussion with Brian Halweil, 1 November 1999; Sweden study from WHO, *Obesity*, op. cit. note 5.

85. WHO, *Obesity*, op. cit. note 5.

86. Neal D. Barnard, Andrew Nicholson, and Jo Lil Howard, "The Medical Costs Attributable to Meat Consumption," *Preventive Medicine*, November 1995.

87. Colditz, op. cit. note 7; $33 billion from Wolf and Colditz, op. cit. note 67.

88. Annual health expenditures per person from Arun Chockalingam and Ignasi Balaguer Vintró, eds., *Impending Global Pandemic of Cardiovascular Diseases* (Barcelona: Prous Science, 1999).

89. WCRF/AICR, op. cit. note 27.

90. Rodolfo A. Bulatao, *The Value of Family Planning Programs in Developing Countries* (Santa Monica, CA: RAND, 1998); WHO, *Obesity*, op. cit. note 5.

91. WHO, op. cit. note 24.

92. Table 6 from Horton, op. cit. note 11.

93. F. James Levinson, "Addressing Malnutrition in Africa," *Social Dimensions of Adjustment In Sub-Saharan Africa*, Working Paper No. 13 (Washington, DC: World Bank, 1991); UN ACC/SCN, op. cit. note 5; Sonya Rabeneck, UN ACC/SCN, e-mail to authors, 10 October 1999; Hanny Friesen, et al., "Protection of Breastfeeding in Papua New Guinea," *Bulletin of the World Health Organization*, vol. 77, no. 3 (1999); Baby-Friendly Hospital Initiative (BFHI) from *BFHI News*, March/April 1999.

94. Marc J. Cohen and Don Reeves, "Causes of Hunger," 2020 Brief 19 (Washington, DC: IFPRI, May 1995); Barbara MkNelly and Christopher Dunford, "Are Credit and Savings Services Effective Against Hunger and Malnutrition?—A Literature Review," Research Paper No. 1 (Davis, CA: Freedom From Hunger, February 1996); IFPRI study from Smith and Haddad, op. cit. note 30.

95. Kerala from C. R. Soman, Professor of Nutrition, College of Medicine,

University of Kerala, e-mail to Brian Halweil, 29 October 1999; Cohen and Reeves, op. cit. note 94.

96. Dotres, op. ct. note 9.

97. Cohen and Reeves, op. cit. note 94; Nancy Birdsall, "Macroeconomic Reform: Its Impact on Poverty and Hunger," in Ismail Serageldin and Pierre Landell-Mills, eds., *Overcoming Global Hunger* (Washington, DC: World Bank, 1993); Per Pinstrup-Andersen and Marc J. Cohen, "Aid to Developing-Country Agriculture: Investing in Poverty Reduction and New Export Opportunities," 2020 Brief 56 (Washington, DC: IFPRI, October 1998).

98. Maurice Schiff and Alberto Valdes, *The Plundering of Agriculture in Developing Countries* (Washington, DC: World Bank, 1992); Lappé, op. cit. note 37.

99. Haddad et al., op. cit. note 18; Catherine Murphy, *Cultivating Havana: Urban Agriculture and Food Security in the Years of Crisis* (Oakland, CA: IFDP, May 1999); share of vegetables from urban gardens from "Cuba Goes Green," *Washington Post*, 26 November 1999.

100. Christopher Dunford, "The Case for Integrated Delivery of Group-based Microfinance Services and Health/Nutrition Behavior Change Education for Cost-Effective Impact on Chronic Food Insecurity and Malnutrition," Freedom from Hunger, draft, 28 May 1999; Barbara MkNelly and Christopher Dunford, "Impact of Credit with Education on Mothers' and Their Young Childrens' Nutrition: Lower Pra Rural Bank Credit with Education Program in Ghana," Research Paper No. 4 (Davis, CA: Freedom from Hunger, March 1998); Muhammad Yunus, "The Grameen Bank," *Scientific American*, November 1999.

101. Ibid.; MkNelly and Dunford, op. cit. note 100.

102. Stuart Gillespie et al., *How Nutrition Improves* (Geneva: WHO, July 1996).

103. Kinday Samba Ndure et al., *Best Practices and Lessons Learned for Sustainable Community Nutrition Programming* (Washington, DC: Academy for Educational Development, August 1999); Josefa S. Eusebio et al., "SAGIP-BATA: BIDANI Strategy for Integrated Household-Based Malnutrition Rehabilitation," Institute of Human Nutrition and Food, University of the Philippines, Los Baños, Philippines, draft.

104. Gillespie et al., op. cit. note 102.

105. Uvin, op. cit. note 37; Pinstrup-Andersen and Cohen, op. cit. note 97; Aileen Kwa, "Will Food Security Get Trampled as the Elephants Fight over Agriculture?" *Focus-on-Trade* No. 36, electronic bulletin from Focus on the Global South, Bangkok, July 1999.

106. Denise Grady, "Doctors' Review of 5 Deaths Raises Concern about the Safety of Liposuction," *New York Times*, 13 May 1999; three common elements from Jane Fritsch, "A Closer Look at Those Who Stay Slim," *New York Times*, 8 June 1999.

107. WHO, *Obesity*, op. cit. note 5; additional Trim and Fit information from Barry M. Popkin, University of North Carolina at Chapel Hill, NC, e-mail to authors, 21 September 1999; U.S. program from P.R. Nader et al., "Three-Year Maintenance of Improved Diet and Physical Activity: The Child and Adolescent Trial for Cardiovascular Health (CATCH) Cohort," *Archives of Pediatrics and Adolescent Medicine*, July 1999.

108. Elizabeth Frazao, ed., op. cit. note 10; Stacey Schultz, "Why We're Fat," *U.S. News & World Report*, 8 November 1999.

109. Meredith May, "Lunch Going Organic, Berkeley Schools to OK Plan for Pesticide-Free Food," *San Francisco Chronicle*, 17 August 1999; Tim Lang, "Get Cooking!" project, National Food Alliance, London, phone conversation with authors, 15 July 1999.

110. Nestle, op. cit. note 42; L.H. Epstein, "Family-based Behavioral Intervention for Obese Children," *International Journal of Obesity Related Metabolic Disorders*, February 1996.

111. C. Howard Davis, "The Report to Congress on the Appropriate Federal Role in Assuring Access by Medical Students, Residents, and Practicing Physicians to Adequate Training in Nutrition," *Public Health Reports*, November/December 1994.

112. Pekka Puska, "Development of Public Policy on the Prevention and Control of Elevated Blood Cholesterol," *Cardiovascular Risk Factors*, August 1996.

113. Consumer survey from *The Shopper Report* (Philadelphia: Consumer Research Network, September 1997).

114. Pekka Puska, "The North Karelia Project: From Community Intervention to National Activity in Lowering Cholesterol Levels and CHD Risk," *European Heart Journal Supplements*, 1999.

115. Tim Lang, "Food & Nutrition in the EU: Its Implications for Public Health," prepared for the European Union Main Public Health Issues Project, September 1998.

116. Kelly D. Brownell, "Get Slim with Higher Taxes," *New York Times*, 15 December 1994.

117. Price change is a Worldwatch calculation from data from the Bureau of Labor Statistics, which uses the consumer price index for the various foods

and compares them to the consumer price index for all foods and beverages.

118. R.W. Jeffrey et al. "An Environmental Intervention to Increase Fruit and Salad Purchases in a Cafeteria," *Preventive Medicine*, November 1994; S.A. French et al., "Pricing Strategy to Promote Low Fat Snack Choices Through Vending Machines," *American Journal of Public Health*, May 1997; S.A. French et al., "Pricing Strategy to Promote Fruit and Vegetable Purchase in High School Cafeterias," *Journal of American Dietetic Association*, September 1997.

119. Slow Food Movement from <www.slowfood.com>, viewed 23 October 1999; Oldways Preservation and Exchange Trust from <www.oldwayspt.org>, viewed 23 October 1999.

120. Nancy Milio, *Nutrition Policy for Food-Rich Countries: A Strategic Analysis* (Baltimore: Johns Hopkins University Press, 1990).

Worldwatch Papers

Worldwatch Papers by Gary Gardner and Brian Halweil

No. of Copies

_____150. **Underfed and Overfed: The Global Epidemic of Malnutrition** by Gary Gardner and Brian Halweil

_____144. **Mind Over Matter: Recasting the Role of Materials in Our Lives** by Gary Gardner and Payal Sampat

_____143. **Beyond Malthus: Sixteen Dimensions of the Population Problem** by Lester R. Brown, Gary Gardner, and Brian Halweil

_____135. **Recycling Organic Waste: From Urban Pollutant to Farm Resource** by Gary Gardner

_____131. **Shrinking Fields: Cropland Loss in a World of Eight Billion** by Gary Gardner

---

_____149. **Paper Cuts: Recovering the Paper Landscape** by Janet N. Abramovitz and Ashley T. Mattoon

_____148. **Nature's Cornucopia: Our Stake in Plant Diversity** by John Tuxill

_____147. **Reinventing Cities for People and the Planet** by Molly O'Meara

_____146. **Ending Violent Conflict** by Michael Renner

_____145. **Safeguarding The Health of Oceans** by Anne Platt McGinn

_____142. **Rocking the Boat: Conserving Fisheries and Protecting Jobs** by Anne Platt McGinn

_____141. **Losing Strands in the Web of Life: Vertebrate Declines and the Conservation of Biological Diversity** by John Tuxill

_____140. **Taking a Stand: Cultivating a New Relationship with the World's Forests** by Janet N. Abramovitz

_____139. **Investing in the Future: Harnessing Private Capital Flows for Environmentally Sustainable Development** by Hilary F. French

_____138. **Rising Sun, Gathering Winds: Policies to Stabilize the Climate and Strengthen Economies** by Christopher Flavin and Seth Dunn

_____137. **Small Arms, Big Impact: The Next Challenge of Disarmament** by Michael Renner

_____136. **The Agricultural Link: How Environmental Deterioration Could Disrupt Economic Progress** by Lester R. Brown

_____134. **Getting the Signals Right: Tax Reform to Protect the Environment and the Economy** by David Malin Roodman

_____133. **Paying the Piper: Subsidies, Politics, and the Environment** by David Malin Roodman

_____132. **Dividing the Waters: Food Security, Ecosystem Health, and the New Politics of Scarcity** by Sandra Postel

_____130. **Climate of Hope: New Strategies for Stabilizing the World's Atmosphere** by Christopher Flavin and Odil Tunali

_____129. **Infecting Ourselves: How Environmental and Social Disruptions Trigger Disease** by Anne E. Platt

_____128. **Imperiled Waters, Impoverished Future: The Decline of Freshwater Ecosystems** by Janet N. Abramovitz

_____127. **Eco-Justice: Linking Human Rights and the Environment** by Aaron Sachs

_____126. **Partnership for the Planet: An Environmental Agenda for the United Nations** by Hilary F. French

_____125. **The Hour of Departure: Forces That Create Refugees and Migrants** by Hal Kane

_____124. **A Building Revolution: How Ecology and Health Concerns Are Transforming Construction** by David Malin Roodman and Nicholas Lenssen

_____123. **High Priorities: Conserving Mountain Ecosystems and Cultures** by Derek Denniston

_____122. **Budgeting for Disarmament: The Costs of War and Peace** by Michael Renner

_____121. **The Next Efficiency Revolution: Creating a Sustainable Materials Economy** by John E. Young and Aaron Sachs

_____**Total copies (transfer number to order form on next page)**

PUBLICATION ORDER FORM

NOTE: Many Worldwatch publications can be downloaded as PDF files from our website at **www.worldwatch.org**. Orders for printed publications can also be placed on the web.

_____ *State of the World:* **$14.95**
The annual book used by journalists, activists, scholars, and policymakers worldwide to get a clear picture of the environmental problems we face.

_____ **State of the World Library: $30.00 (international subscribers $45)**
Receive *State of the World* and all five Worldwatch Papers as they are released during the calendar year.

_____ *Vital Signs:* **$13.00**
The book of trends that are shaping our future in easy-to-read graph and table format, with a brief commentary on each trend.

_____ **WORLD WATCH magazine subscription: $20.00 (international airmail $35.00)**
Stay abreast of global environmental trends and issues with our award-winning, eminently readable bimonthly magazine.

_____ **Worldwatch Database Disk Subscription: $89.00**
Contains global agricultural, energy, economic, environmental, social, and military indicators from all current Worldwatch publications. Includes a mid-year update, and *Vital Signs* and *State of the World* as they are published. Disk contains Microsoft Excel spreadsheets 5.0/95 (*.xls) for Windows.
Check one: ____ **PC** ____ **Mac**

_____ **Worldwatch Papers—See list on previous page**
Single copy: $5.00
2–5: $4.00 ea. • 6–20: $3.00 ea. • 21 or more: $2.00 ea.

$4.00* Shipping and Handling *($8.00 outside North America)*
*minimum charge for S&H; call (800) 555-2028 for bulk order S&H

_____ **TOTAL** (U.S. dollars only)

Make check payable to: Worldwatch Institute, 1776 Massachusetts Ave., NW, Washington, DC 20036-1904 USA

Enclosed is my check or purchase order for U.S. $_____

☐ AMEX ☐ VISA ☐ MasterCard _____
Card Number   Expiration Date

_____
signature

_____
name   **daytime phone #**

_____
address

_____
city   **state**   **zip/country**

phone: (800) 555-2028   fax: (202) 296-7365   e-mail: wwpub@worldwatch.org
website: www.worldwatch.org

Wish to make a tax-deductible contribution? Contact Worldwatch to find out how your donation can help advance our work.

Worldwatch Papers

Worldwatch Papers by Gary Gardner and Brian Halweil

No. of Copies

_____150. **Underfed and Overfed: The Global Epidemic of Malnutrition** by Gary Gardner and
Brian Halweil

_____144. **Mind Over Matter: Recasting the Role of Materials in Our Lives**
by Gary Gardner and Payal Sampat

_____143. **Beyond Malthus: Sixteen Dimensions of the Population Problem**
by Lester R. Brown, Gary Gardner, and Brian Halweil

_____135. **Recycling Organic Waste: From Urban Pollutant to Farm Resource** by Gary Gardner

_____131. **Shrinking Fields: Cropland Loss in a World of Eight Billion** by Gary Gardner

_____149. **Paper Cuts: Recovering the Paper Landscape** by Janet N. Abramovitz
and Ashley T. Mattoon

_____148. **Nature's Cornucopia: Our Stake in Plant Diversity** by John Tuxill

_____147. **Reinventing Cities for People and the Planet** by Molly O'Meara

_____146. **Ending Violent Conflict** by Michael Renner

_____145. **Safeguarding The Health of Oceans** by Anne Platt McGinn

_____142. **Rocking the Boat: Conserving Fisheries and Protecting Jobs** by Anne Platt McGinn

_____141. **Losing Strands in the Web of Life: Vertebrate Declines and the Conservation of
Biological Diversity** by John Tuxill

_____140. **Taking a Stand: Cultivating a New Relationship with the World's Forests**
by Janet N. Abramovitz

_____139. **Investing in the Future: Harnessing Private Capital Flows for Environmentally
Sustainable Development** by Hilary F. French

_____138. **Rising Sun, Gathering Winds: Policies to Stabilize the Climate and Strengthen
Economies** by Christopher Flavin and Seth Dunn

_____137. **Small Arms, Big Impact: The Next Challenge of Disarmament** by Michael Renner

_____136. **The Agricultural Link: How Environmental Deterioration Could Disrupt Economic
Progress** by Lester R. Brown

_____134. **Getting the Signals Right: Tax Reform to Protect the Environment and the Economy**
by David Malin Roodman

_____133. **Paying the Piper: Subsidies, Politics, and the Environment** by David Malin Roodman

_____132. **Dividing the Waters: Food Security, Ecosystem Health, and the New Politics of
Scarcity** by Sandra Postel

_____130. **Climate of Hope: New Strategies for Stabilizing the World's Atmosphere**
by Christopher Flavin and Odil Tunali

_____129. **Infecting Ourselves: How Environmental and Social Disruptions Trigger
Disease** by Anne E. Platt

_____128. **Imperiled Waters, Impoverished Future: The Decline of Freshwater Ecosystems**
by Janet N. Abramovitz

_____127. **Eco-Justice: Linking Human Rights and the Environment** by Aaron Sachs

_____126. **Partnership for the Planet: An Environmental Agenda for the United Nations**
by Hilary F. French

_____125. **The Hour of Departure: Forces That Create Refugees and Migrants** by Hal Kane

_____124. **A Building Revolution: How Ecology and Health Concerns Are Transforming
Construction** by David Malin Roodman and Nicholas Lenssen

_____123. **High Priorities: Conserving Mountain Ecosystems and Cultures**
by Derek Denniston

_____122. **Budgeting for Disarmament: The Costs of War and Peace** by Michael Renner

_____121. **The Next Efficiency Revolution: Creating a Sustainable Materials Economy**
by John E. Young and Aaron Sachs

_____**Total copies (transfer number to order form on next page)**

PUBLICATION ORDER FORM

NOTE: Many Worldwatch publications can be downloaded as PDF files from our website at **www.worldwatch.org**. Orders for printed publications can also be placed on the web.

_____ *State of the World:* **$14.95**
   The annual book used by journalists, activists, scholars, and policymakers worldwide to get a clear picture of the environmental problems we face.

_____ **State of the World Library: $30.00 (international subscribers $45)**
   Receive *State of the World* and all five Worldwatch Papers as they are released during the calendar year.

_____ *Vital Signs:* **$13.00**
   The book of trends that are shaping our future in easy-to-read graph and table format, with a brief commentary on each trend.

_____ **WORLD WATCH magazine subscription: $20.00 (international airmail $35.00)**
   Stay abreast of global environmental trends and issues with our award-winning, eminently readable bimonthly magazine.

_____ **Worldwatch Database Disk Subscription: $89.00**
   Contains global agricultural, energy, economic, environmental, social, and military indicators from all current Worldwatch publications. Includes a mid-year update, and *Vital Signs* and *State of the World* as they are published. Disk contains Microsoft Excel spreadsheets 5.0/95 (*.xls) for Windows.
   Check one: _____ **PC** _____ **Mac**

_____ **Worldwatch Papers—See list on previous page**
   Single copy: $5.00
   2–5: $4.00 ea. • 6–20: $3.00 ea. • 21 or more: $2.00 ea.

$4.00* Shipping and Handling *($8.00 outside North America)*
   *minimum charge for S&H; call (800) 555-2028 for bulk order S&H

_____ **TOTAL** (U.S. dollars only)

Make check payable to: Worldwatch Institute, 1776 Massachusetts Ave., NW, Washington, DC 20036-1904 USA

Enclosed is my check or purchase order for U.S. $_____

☐ AMEX ☐ VISA ☐ MasterCard _____
                                   Card Number   Expiration Date

_____
signature

_____
name   **daytime phone #**

_____
address

_____
city   **state**   **zip/country**

phone: (800) 555-2028   fax: (202) 296-7365   e-mail: wwpub@worldwatch.org
website: www.worldwatch.org

Wish to make a tax-deductible contribution? Contact Worldwatch to find out how your donation can help advance our work.

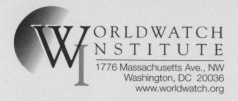

WORLDWATCH INSTITUTE

1776 Massachusetts Ave., NW
Washington, DC 20036
www.worldwatch.org

WORLDWATCH PAPER 150

Underfed and Overfed: The Global Epidemic of Malnutrition

Three billion people—more than half of the global population—are malnourished, suffering from hunger, vitamin and mineral deficiency, or overeating. And for the first time in history the world's overweight population now rivals the number that is underweight.

The hungry and the overweight often face similar impairments: increased risk of disease and disability, reduced productivity, and reduced life expectancy. The World Bank estimates that hunger cost India between 3 and 9 percent of its GDP in 1996, while obesity cost the United States $118 billion—some 12 percent of what the nation spends on health care. For individuals as well as societies, malnutrition is a drag on development.

But the reverse is also true: poor development choices spawn malnourished societies. Where hunger is the problem, governments have often failed to assure access to land and other productive resources, as well as basic social services. Where overeating is the issue, policymakers have typically neglected nutrition education, allowing giant food companies to influence people's food choices by default.

In an age of unprecedented wealth, there is no excuse for malnutrition on such a massive scale. From the Indian state of Kerala to the island of Singapore, governments that appreciate the role of nutrition in national development and make good nutrition a priority demonstrate that both hunger and obesity can largely be eliminated.